A Change of Heart

Journal of a Heart Transplant

Bill Long

The Cardiac Surgical Foundation

Heart disease is the single most common type of fatal illness in Ireland today. Most heart diseases can be corrected using modern surgical techniques. And yet there are over sixteen hundred people in the country awaiting Cardiac Surgery, waiting for the chance to live their lives fully once more

The Cardiac Surgical Foundation is about self-help. Its mission is to create the circumstances in which everybody, irrespective of ability to pay, can have life-saving cardiac surgery. It hopes to raise five million pounds to increase the number of operating theatres in the public sector, which would substantially increase the country's cardiac surgical capabilities.

For more information please contact The Cardiac Surgical Foundation, by telephone at 01-6685699 or by post at 114 Pembroke Road, Dublin 4.

Maurice Neligan,
Director,
The Cardiac Surgical Foundation.

A
Change
of
Heart

Journal of a Heart Transplant

Bill Long

New Island Books / Dublin

A Change of Heart
is first published in 1995 by
New Island Books,
2, Brookside,
Dundrum Road,
Dublin 14,
Ireland

ISBN 1 874597 21 9

New Island Books receives financial assistance from
The Arts Council (An Chomhairle Ealaíon),
Dublin, Ireland.

Cover photo of Bill Long at the Baily lighthouse by
Derek Speirs
Cover design by Jon Berkeley
Typeset by Graphic Resources
Printed in Ireland by Colour Books, Ltd.

Dedicated to Maurice Neligan, Brian Maurer and my donor.

" Well, World, you have kept faith with me,
 Kept faith with me;
Upon the whole you have proved to be
 Much as you said you were.
Since as a child I used to lie
 Upon the leaze and watch the sky,
Never, I own, expected I
 That life would all be fair."

Thomas Hardy: 'He Never Expected Much'

Introduction

This journal was begun in late January 1994, on the day when I was told I must have a heart transplant. The initial motivation was selfish; a need to rationalise the shock news for myself by verbalising it on paper. In the crises and traumas of my life I have always turned first to my typewriter, as others might to their psychiatrist. I have found it to be my best 'shrink'. But, only if I am totally honest in what I write; only if, metaphorically speaking, I take my clothes off in public and step out, with as much abandon as I can muster, onto the tight-rope, having eschewed the insurance of the safety-net.

This worked well for me. Inside a week I had come to terms with my condition, had begun to assimilate the enormity of what lay ahead, and had begun to learn how to cope with the mood swings, the good days and the bad. By then, from my observations of my fellow-patients in the Intensive Care Unit of Coronary Care, another motive, totally selfless this time, had presented itself as added justification for writing the journal. I saw so many people, some much younger than myself, who couldn't cope with the news that they needed heart surgery; not necessarily transplant, but by-pass or relatively simple angioplasty. They became traumatised for days, refusing to talk to anyone, even their closest family and dearest friends. And watching this temporary exclusion of those closest to them, I experienced something of their trauma too; wondering if the surgery would be successful; wondering how they would cope with the waiting and the convalescence. The journal might help such people; not just those needing heart transplant, but anyone, patient or care-giver, faced with the trauma of any major surgery.

Then, as my long wait for the new heart stretched from weeks into months, and I spent most of the warm summer, like a recidivist prisoner, in and out of hospital, a third motive became very obvious. The need for more organ donors. I saw this as a very urgent pre-requisite after my pre-operative meetings with Mr Maurice Neligan and his team. If people like myself were to survive, then more donors must be forthcoming. So, the journal might help raise the level of public awareness to the vital importance of donorship; not just heart, but general organ donorship. It might remind people that, for those like myself, whose heart, liver or kidneys had all but totally failed, there was no hope without the charity, love and magnanimity of the donor. For me there was the daily nightmare of wondering which would come first, the fatal attack or the new heart; a kind of Russian Roulette.

And then there was the surgery itself. The new heart, like a visitor long awaited, surprising me in the end by the suddenness, the arbitrariness of its arrival. That, and the trauma of intensive care and subsequent recuperation gave added validity to the project. There were many things people could learn from my experience. I remembered, every day, what the English novelist John Fowles said of honesty of expression: "The writer is like a man on a tight-rope. He must balance and he must move." I hope I have succeeded in keeping my equilibrium through the good days and the bad, maintained some grace under pressure, and leavened it all with some sense of humour, even some sense of the ridiculous. For, often, in traumatic, life-threatening situations, a sense of humour is not enough; we need a sense of the ridiculous to see us through.

But, more than all that; more than the courage and the faith, the sense of humour or of the ridiculous, we need the humility, in such extremities, to abandon ourselves to some Power greater than ourselves. A Power that holds us all in the hollow of Its benign hand and disposes of our various destinies. Call it what you will, according to your particular belief, or unbelief; the Gods, the Fates, Jesus, Buddha, Nada. For, in addition to the magnanimous donor and the expert and caring medical team, we need a certain element of miracle, with a small 'm'. And, only with the humility of abandonment can the miracle begin.

Bill Long
28th April 1995

PART ONE:

At Hazard

"Does the road wind uphill all the way?
Yes, to the very end.
Will the day's journey take the whole long day?
From morn to night, my friend."

Christina Rossetti: 'Up-Hill'

Late January 1994. The real dead-end of the year. My hospital bed is beside a large picture-window and I can see the sickly, yellowish light filtered through the scudding sheets of bruise-grey rain-cloud. The great grove of old trees across the lawn is a skeletal, twisted black trellis against the unrelieved drab backdrop of the swollen sky. But, my spirits are relatively high this morning. It's been two days since my last attack, and I am recovering some strength and free of pain. This may be, despite the weather, a good day. I have an ambition for today. A modest ambition, relatively speaking, for, after four weeks of hospitalisation, everything one does, or plans to do, becomes relative. Today, after nearly a week of being confined to bed and having to use bed pan and urinal bottle, I am hopeful I shall be allowed to walk out to the toilet, which is only ten yards down the corridor. Such a walk would help restore my dented dignity, make me feel less bed-ridden and useless.

Mirrored in the big window is the usual flux of white-uniformed figures, nurses and doctors, coming and going in the ward. One white figure detaches itself from the rest and comes toward my bed. I leave my contemplation of the scene outside my window and turn to see who it is. It is the Senior Staff Sister and she brings a chair and sits beside me. Usually she stands. She talks about the result of my angiogram. The grafts from my quadruple by-pass of eight years ago are not, as was suspected, the problem. The problem is cardiomyopathy, a disease of the muscle of the heart, which, unfortunately, can neither be arrested nor repaired. Transplant, it seems, is the only answer. Sister explains that Dr Brian Maurer, the Consultant Cardiologist, will be coming to talk to me about the details later. Before she leaves I ask her what can have caused my condition; I have been so careful about food, drink, exercise, since my by-pass surgery. She smiles and says: "It's usually caused by a biochemical defect or excessive use of alcohol." I laugh through the chaos of my feelings and assure her that in my case it's certainly not alcohol!

After she has gone I am in a state of shock, devastated. For, badly as I had been feeling since Christmas, I had thought my condition might be managed with medication or rectified with angioplasty or further by-pass. Transplant had never occurred to me. The concept seems unreal, outlandish. I am totally confused, struggle to grasp or accept it. And, as often happens in moments of shock or crisis, one focuses on some detail of what happens to be in one's immediate vision at that moment and remembers it forever. Like the gravy, heavy and dead and brown, coagulating in its 'boat' on the dinner table, when you were eleven or twelve and had just been severely reprimanded, on some special occasion, for your abominable table manners. Or the colour, and number, and exact shape and symmetry of the rungs of the old iron gate, where you stood, under the winter stars in freezing cold, and had your first serious row with your first serious girl-friend.

Turning again to the scene outside my window, my eyes do not go directly to the dark, trellised trees or the bruise-grey sky, but to the wide lawn where two magpies strut and hop in loud, cacophonous glee, round a hedgehog slowly moving toward the copse. They immediately become my focus in crisis, etched in my memory forever, synonymous with heart transplant. For that is all I can think of now. My head aches and the two terrible syllables...'trans - plant'...ring like hammer on anvil in my mind. One part of me calmly watches the antics of the hedgehog and the magpies; another part of me is in shock. My simple ambition for the day — to go out to the toilet — is quickly forgotten and I am calling nurse to get me the urine bottle. When she brings it and asks if I need the curtain drawn, I say "No, thank you." It is that quiet time of mid-morning; rounds are over and there are no visitors yet. My fellow-patients are reading or dozing. There is something claustro-phobic about curtains drawn round the bed. Still in a state of shock I slip the bottle under the bedclothes and begin to urinate. And, for the first time ever, I am hyper-conscious of the noise. What is, in reality, the gentle trickle of water into the urinal becomes the tumbling of a mountain stream in spate. I steal a glance at my fellow patients. The dozers are still dozing, the readers still reading. They, obviously, have not heard the roar of the waters. Desperately, I will them to remain that way, and in my desperation I freeze the first image, the first thought, that comes into my mind. It is of the 'darksome burn' described in Gerard Manley Hopkins' poem 'Inversnaid'. One of my favourite poems. I know it well, and quickly, silently, I begin to repeat it, a rune against my fellow-patients hearing:

This darksome burn, horseback brown,

His rollrock highroad roaring down,

In coop and in comb the fleece of his foam

Flutes and low to the lake falls home.

A windpuff-bonnet of fawn-froth

Turns and twindles over the broth

Of a pool so pitchback, fell frowning,

It rounds and rounds Despair to drowning.

Degged with dew, dappled with dew

Are the groins of the braes that the brook treads through...

This line about 'the groins of the braes' breaks me up, jolts me out of my state of shock, and makes me think of the plastic bottle between my legs and of how ludicrous it is to be even concerned about the trickle of water, barely audible, under the bedclothes. And I go, instantly, from the sublime to the ridiculous. My mind jumps from the beautiful Hopkins poem to remembering an incident in a small hotel in Cavan some years ago. I found myself in the toilet, standing side by side at the urinals with a farmer whose son had gone into one of the cubicles and left the door open. As they urinated they carried on a conversation about the wedding they were attending. Both were inebriated. They fell silent when I entered and in the silence the son's urinating into the toilet bowl sounded like the rains of Ranchipur in monsoon season. Without looking at me the old man said, very politely: "Excuse him, sir, he's at a weddin'." As I left, he shouted at the son: "God! Have ye no manners? Couldn't ye side it a bit and not make so much shaggin' noise!" The memory of this makes me laugh outright, which rouses some of my dozing companions and causes my next-door-neighbour to abandon his reading. He and I have been neighbours for two weeks and shared many a joke, in good times and bad. He looks at me quizzically and asks: "Ah, a new joke! Don't hold out on us. Let's have it!" And with tears in my

11

eyes, tears of laughter and tears of confusion, I answer, with as much casualness as I can muster: "Why not. I'm going to have a heart transplant."

□□□

The sleepers are not roused, bandaged by sleep against my laughter. The readers put down their books and papers and magazines and stare at me silently. They are shocked, as I am. It takes them a few minutes to react, and their reaction is predictable; for the very ill, as we all are here in Intensive Care, invariably show a positive attitude at such times. While the whole concept of transplant may be shocking, the alternative is totally insuperable. So, they put a brave face on things, as much for themselves as for me and, with a fine bravado, offer well-meant comforting platitudes like: "Well, aren't you lucky to be getting a new heart." "Isn't it great you're a suitable subject for transplant; not everyone is." "You'll have a new lease of life." They even joke about "the old engine being rebored and good for another hundred thousand miles." One patient who, more than the others, appreciates my sense of the ridiculous, even jokes about the possibility of my getting a female heart. "I'll never know whose heart I get," I retort. "Oh, but you will," he says, "when your voice changes and goes all falsetto and you start hitting people with your handbag."

But soon the badinage, the humour, the glib, well-intentioned remarks, become forced and we all lapse into silence again; each one of us locked into his own strait-jacket of illness, doubt and apprehension. We are like survivors of a sinking ship, floundering now in deep waters, desperately clinging to the wreckage of battered life-boats and splintered spars. So, we let the silence wash over us, each one of us lost now in his own personal kingdom of memory and imagination, but still hyper-sensitive to each other's condition. For, within the narrow world of this Coronary Care Unit, no man is an island. We are all here with defective hearts. One man's problem is each man's problem. With the awful arbitrariness of heart disease what happens to one this morning may happen to another this afternoon. One picks up again his Financial Times, but without much real interest now in the fluctuations of the stock market. Another reads, without much enthusiasm, his daily newspaper. A third returns to his scrofulous American novel with far less relish than when he put it down. Another replaces his headphones and tries to lose himself in the majestic swell of Beethoven's music.

❏❏❏

For myself, I lie here and gaze again at the scene outside my window. The sky is clearing, great shining patches of bright blue predominating. The clouds are rolling away before a wind from the west and the bare trees look less gaunt and black. The wind is visible in the short winter grass, flattening it, riffling it. Though the hedgehog has long since made his escape into the undergrowth, the two marauding magpies, silent now, but obviously still hopeful, stand guard at the edge of the copse. And I think of the long-ago time, when my children were small, babies in their prams on the back lawn, and I would regularly have to go out and chase the cheeky, raucous magpies away. I remember a line from a poem, or piece of prose, that described the magpie, with his long, narrow tail and wide wings, as 'a flying frying pan'. I try to remember who wrote that, but can't. Could have been Dylan Thomas. I am not sure. Away down the long corridor outside the ward I can hear the rumble of the lunch-trolley and the clatter of the plates. I try to remember what I've ordered for lunch, but can't. Part of me is still numb. The lunch trolley reminds me of the other trolley I've heard once come in the night: to take the body away when someone has died of heart failure. I lie back on my pillows and weep.

❏❏❏

Why do I weep? I weep because I am afraid. Afraid of what? Afraid of Death? No. Not so much afraid of Death as afraid of the loss of Life. The Life that, until now, I thought stretched endlessly before me, offering me ample time in which to write all the things I want to write. Now, with this transplant, and, to my confused and unenlightened mind, the possible serious, or perhaps fatal consequences, I can see that time slipping away, while I lie helplessly here. Eventually, I dry my tears and try to eat some lunch.

❏❏❏

Outside my window the stark and sombre outline of the skeletal trees is relieved by slanting sunset light. Through the lower branches I can see the last players dotted round the adjoining golf course, like tiny coloured patches glowing in the near-dusk. How I envy those winter golfers! And, what I envy most about them is their mobility. Watching them from my position of total immobility in this hospital bed, their

13

every movement seems exaggerated; the practice swings, the endless shifting of stance as they address the ball, the ease with which they haul their caddy-cars. It seems incredible to me that four months ago I was playing golf, so devoid am I now of any spark of energy. It seems equally incredible that I'll ever be well enough to play golf again. The thought of taking a club in my hands, flexing it, swinging it high above my shoulders and then bringing it down and through the ball, fills me with near panic. After this last attack I find it difficult to even hold a comb and raise my hand above my head to comb my hair. How much worse will it be after transplant surgery, I ask myself, in my ignorance. I am terribly tense and negative about it all. Negative to the point of being defeatist.

After tea I am a little less tense; relaxed enough to read my, as yet unopened, morning paper. It is all mayhem, war and politics. Murder, rape, drug-abuse, robbery, fraud, litigation of one nasty kind or other, steal the headlines on every page. The 'Comment' columns proliferate. Every columnist is an expert on everything. There are endless analyses, endless definitive statements, endless remedies, yet nothing is ever remedied. It is as if some film has been peeled from my eyes; some screen, that heretofore has kept me from a real appreciation of the craziness of the world, removed. Nothing like a bit of shock news to change one's perspective, make one appreciate how relative everything is. Yesterday other peoples' problems were of some interest to me; today they are not. The only problem I am aware of today is my own. For the moment every man is an island. This is my life on the line in this transplant operation. Even my fellow patients, with whom I have the common bond of heart disease have, temporarily at least, ceased to interest me. Later, when I've come to terms with my predicament, I am to feel very shamefaced about my selfishness, but now I am shocked, confused, and wait the visit of Dr Brian Maurer, my Cardiologist...

Brian Maurer, Consultant Cardiologist at St. Vincent's Hospital is an extraordinary man; a man in whom there is such a felicitous conjunction of energy, tenderness, pragmatism, caring, wisdom and diagnostic expertise. Nine years ago his perspicacity and quick action saved my life. I had just suffered two severe heart attacks then, within a few days. While others pondered what action to take, he, quickly assessing the gravity of my condition, sent me for emergency cardiac surgery. I have no doubt that the quadruple by-pass saved my life. I trust him implicitly. Sitting here waiting for him to arrive, I feel a growing certainty that, despite my ignorance of any detail of the heart transplant procedure, if he has recommended it, I must accept it as the best thing for me. So, when he comes, pulls the curtain and sits on the side of my bed, I have made up my mind. Before he can tell me anything I find myself saying, quite calmly, as if I had just made a decision, without even looking at the menu, to accept the recommendation of the maitre d' in a good restaurant — "I've decided to have it. Now, please, tell me all about it." Putting his hand on my shoulder, he answers me with reassuring equanimity: "I think you have made the absolutely right decision. I'll set the wheels in motion right away and arrange an appointment with Maurice Neligan." Then, without further preamble he proceeds to tell me why, and how and where. When cannot be forecast; that depends on many factors beyond his, or my control; principally the availability and suitability of a donor heart.

□□□

Brian Maurer explains that my cardiomyopathy is a direct result of the serious damage caused to my heart muscle when I suffered the two attacks nine years ago. There is no reversing the condition, no way of repairing it; my condition will deteriorate steadily, and as the muscle gets weaker I will find it increasingly difficult to breathe, with a consequent serious curtailment of any kind of physical activity. More and more rest will be mandatory; as much as twenty hours a day. More and more medication will be essential to preserve the tentative pulse of life and conserve the little energy I am now capable of generating. And, despite all the rest and the medication, the quality of my life will steadily deteriorate. I tell him I am already aware of this deterioration; walking is difficult, talking is difficult. Every movement, however slight, however economical, saps that minimal energy. Indeed, often, just resting, I gasp for breath. My breathing is becoming such a problem that soon I won't be able to broadcast or lecture anymore. He promises to stress the urgency of my need for a new heart when he talks with Maurice Neligan later this week. Meantime, he will do everything he can to make me as comfortable as possible. He will arrange a special medication programme for me. One of his senior registrars will supervise this. After we have talked for ten minutes it is all said. Brian Maurer and myself are both people who know when to get off the phone, who know that any further talk is going to be just repetition, So, with a silent smile and a firm hand-clasp Brian Maurer leaves me. I motion to him as he goes not to pull back the curtains. I have a great need to be left alone.

❏❏❏

I am allowed out of bed this morning, for the first time in ten days. It is untold joy to sit beside the window and read and write, free of the harness of wires and tubes from monitors and drips. I am writing some pieces for 'Sunday Miscellany', the Irish radio 'Music and Musings' programme to which I have been contributing for the past eight years. Lorelei Harris, the producer, has suggested that my friend John MacKenna should read them for me. My breathing is too laboured to read anything myself. I have tried recording them, here in the ward, but the result is certainly not suitable for public broadcasting. But my joy changes to depression as I look at my Marantz Recording unit with its scuffed and travel-stained case, and think of the hundreds of people I have recorded on it for the many documentaries I've made. It's travelled with me all over Ireland, to Wales, to London, and to Central America. Now, I feel I shall never use it again. For it seems inconceivable that I shall ever have enough strength to pack a bag and travel again; even go into studio again and record a five-minute talk. That part of my life seems to have fallen into the sea and disappeared, like some ruined tower on a headland eroded by the waves. I finish the piece I am writing and feel so despondent that I cannot start the second piece. I spend the rest of the morning wallowing in self-pity. By lunchtime I have decided that self-pity is futile, a total waste of time. I resolve to eat a good lunch, take my usual afternoon nap and, on waking, be positive and start work again.

❏❏❏

I wake, in mid-afternoon, from a dream so graphic and real that for a little while I am totally disorientated. The ward, the monitors above the beds, the blinds lowered against the afternoon sun, my sleeping fellow-patients, the nurse sitting at a small table filling in reports, are all unreal. I ask myself how I got here. For the dreamland from which I've just returned was very different. In it I sat on the balcony of 'The Boathouse' at Laugharne, and drank wine with Dylan Thomas, Raymond Chandler, Henry Miller and Thomas Merton. An enormous dish of fresh prawns, still in the shell, stood in the centre of the table.

Each of us helped himself, shelling the prawns and throwing the shells on the floor, where they had built up into a flamingo pink mound. At intervals Dylan's daughter, Aeron, a chubby girl of seven or eight, came from the house with more wine. A golden-coloured Shetland collie dog nosed about the pile of discarded shells, sniffing them, attempting to lick off the tiny particles of meat still adhering to them. But, the shells kept sticking to his tongue. He coughed, and spluttered and whined disconsolately and then went away. It was ebb-tide, and the golden sands of the estuary stretched away to the thin, blue line of the water over against the far shore. Cockle-pickers, in little groups, bent to their task, black and small as birds, far out near the tide's edge. Garrulous gulls squabbled as they strutted and fished the shallow pools left by the ebbed tide; a raucous cacophony of crows flew home to Sir John's Hill across the horseshoe bay. Sheer above us the summer sunlight drowned in the lush-foliaged trees overhanging the cliff-walk. Invisible birds sang sweetly in their branches. Faintly, in the distance, the town-hall clock in Laugharne struck three. Dylan, wine glass in one hand, cigarette in the other, recited some lines from his poem, 'Fern Hill':

> And then to awake, and the farm, like a wanderer white
> With the dew, come back, the cock on his shoulder: it was all
> Shining, it was Adam and maiden...

And, in the dream, Merton immediately took issue with Dylan as to how he had read the poem; objecting to the "booming and bazooming" voice. Thomas, aggrieved and argumentative, retorted that it was "his poem and he would read it whatever way he fucking well liked." Miller and Chandler, chewed their prawns, sipped their wine and smiled in anticipation of a good fiery argument. Then, as with all interesting dreams, just when something exciting was about to happen, it ended.

□□□

I sit on my bed, the late afternoon sun full on the window beside me, and ruminate on my dream. I don't dream very often, but when I do there are always 'connections' in the dream. By that I mean the dream always reflects, in however direct or indirect a way, something from my past, or presages something in my future. There are always 'connections' between the ostensibly disparate elements of the dream, and identifying these 'connections' is always a stimulating, sometimes pleasant, sometimes disturbing, exercise. And this dream of four writers, all dead, chewing prawns and sipping wine with me on a balcony above an ebbed sea in a remote corner of Wales, is a classic example of the subtle alchemy these 'connections' can weave in the subconscious, drawing all those diverse threads together, transmuting everything into a mesmeric chiaroscuro of images and sounds.

Sitting here analysing this dream is very much more pleasant than disturbing. For, really, there is very little in it of fantasy. It is almost all based on 'facts', as they happened in my past. But the 'facts' have been taken and reworked in the fire of some benevolent, divine imagination; all the 'connections' made, all the visuals enhanced, all the aural effects heightened. It only remains for me to recognise those 'connections'. The only one of the four I have never met is Dylan Thomas; but I have met his daughter, Aeron; not as the little girl in my dream, but as a woman of fifty, when she and I made a radio documentary about her father. In that programme she talked about her father, when she was seven or eight, and his great love of Raymond Chandler's detective stories. And, in the time I knew Merton, in the 1960s, during his last years at Gethsemani, he spoke often about the importance of Dylan as the great lyric poet of our time, and wrote a long poem, 'Sports Without Blood', for Dylan Thomas. Miller had, when I met him in New York, also in the 1960s, begun a correspondence with Merton. The two, almost diametrically opposed on many things, thought highly of each other's work and, despite irreconcilably differing viewpoints, respected each other greatly; proving Merton's dictum that we were "all born under the same sign, the sign of contradiction." The dog in my dream was my own collie, Pepe, who, coincidentally, had fallen ill about the same time I did. After twelve years his heart, kidneys and prostate had begun to fail, and his slow deterioration was being carefully attended and monitored by a very solicitous vet. As always with dreams, when I pass them through this fire of memory and imagination, they yield up these 'connections' I had not thought existed, or had all but forgotten. Like some miraculous X-ray picture revealing the subtle secrets under the skin; the arteries and the tributary veins, the bones and the sinews, that constitute the tell-tale map.

❏❏❏

Just after midnight. The ward is quiet, lit only by the dim night-light set into the wall beside the open door, the faint over-spill of light from the corridor, and the flickering traceries of the monitors above each bed. One by one the late night readers have switched off their bedside lamps and are sleeping now. A couple of the snorers have already begun to limber up for a heavy snoring session, their intermittent grunts and groans, snorts and snuffles desecrating the silence, warning of the thunder to come. The blinds are down on all the windows and I can hear the trees sway and creak in the wicked February wind. From the relative safety and comfort of this hospital bed the wind seems to me a living thing, prowling about the lawn, soughing and sighing in the bare trees and the little copse. And, when, momentarily, it gusts to gale force, rattling the windows, it sounds like a donkey rubbing its haunches against the glass. It is difficult to believe that we are already nearly a week into spring. The heating is on, but the night-air is chill. In the corridor, directly in front of the entrance to the ward, the night-nurse has set up a trolley and chair and is busy filling out her reports. The corridor is a draughty place and she has wrapped a blanket round her lower body to protect her legs and feet. She is no older than my youngest daughter. Watching her I listen to the great wash of wind outside my window and try to remember the Robert Louis Stevenson poem about the night-horseman... *"All night long in the dark and wet a man goes riding by ..."* But, disorientated by the medication I have taken just a few hours ago, I cannot remember any more of the poem I read so often to my children when they were small. Even with the help of a sleeping pill I cannot sleep. Not so much cannot, as will not, for I am afraid some nights to go to sleep. Stricken with an inordinate, irrational fear that, if I go to sleep I will not waken again. Fearful that a new heart attack will ambush me and take me, unaware. So, with a great pragmatism, in an effort to break this circuit of fear and sleeplessness, I get out of bed and put on dressing-gown and slippers and go to the toilet. The night-nurse smiles at me as I pass and whispers: "Would you like a cup of tea?" I return her smile and nod, "Yes, please!" A little later, when she takes the tea to my bedside, one of the snorers has wakened suddenly. I can see him sitting bolt upright in the semi-darkness, huffing and puffing like a man who has just surfaced from deep water. Nurse whispers something to him as she goes out and returns with a cup of tea for him also. We finish our tea and wave silently to each other, before sinking down again behind the dim, white horizons of our respective counterpanes to, hopefully, drift into sleep.

This morning I have just set myself up to write when nurse comes and announces a visitor. It is Dermot Bolger, my publisher, hirsute and jovial who brings the good news that my book, *Bright Light, White Water*, has sold well over Christmas. Characteristically he twines the end of his long beard round his forefinger and asks what I am writing now.

"Just a note-book, a kind of journal, to rationalise this transplant business and help me stay sane."

"Great. I'll publish it when you're over your transplant and fully recovered."

"But what if I don't recover, don't get over the surgery?"

"I'll still publish it. Probably sell more copies if you don't!"

We both laugh. We understand each other perfectly. Others might not. We both appreciate that there are some situations so critical that a mere sense of humour is not enough in dealing with them. One needs a sense of the ridiculous.

I introduce Dermot to Dr Maurer. "You must look after this man," Dermot tells him, "he can't die yet. He's got a contract with me for two more books."

❏❏❏

The second week in February. From my hospital bed I am aware of the first, tentative intimations and inventions of spring. The immemorial trees are still bare, but now there is a suggestion of the beginnings of tiny buds swelling along their branches. In the copse under the trees there is just the subtlest hint of colour among the various flowering shrubs and bushes; as if some sublime watercolourist had deftly applied the faintest wash of green. An almost imperceptible, luminous patina, perhaps only visible to the very ill. For, I look on everything now as if I shall never see it again, my perceptions heightened by the presence of the killer in my chest. Along the skirts of the copse a dim, white dust of snowdrops, like muted footlights in a theatre, waiting to come up full on some major production. And, here and there, not in formal beds, but randomly, growing directly out of the grass, little clumps of daffodils. Some of the blooms still folded tight in the green bulging heads; others, full blown, loud yellow trumpets sounding the retreat of winter, heralding the charge of spring. Unbidden, Swinburne's lovely lines come to my mind, albeit in fits and starts, my memory blurred by the heavy medication:

When the hounds of Spring are on Winter's traces,
The mother of months in meadow and plain
Fills the shadows and windy places
With lisp of leaves and ripple of rain...

The rest is beyond my remembering, all except one line. One sad, beautiful, and, for me, partly apposite line... *"The tongueless vigil, and all the pain."* I say partly, because my vigil, though pain-filled, is not entirely tongueless. This journal I write is my tongue. My stammering, faltering, boisterous, gentle, contradictory, inconsistent, irreverent and elliptical tongue.

□□□

Monday next will be Valentine's Day. Already the newspapers, radio, television, are full of vulgar commercial hype. My daughter and her boyfriend have just been to visit me, enthusing about how they are going to celebrate it. For myself it will be a bonus to be still alive, and a double-bonus to be pain free, as I have now for nearly a week. After a period of trial with my medication I am now what is termed 'stabilised'. This means a 'diet' of six different medications; tablets, capsules, liquids, three times a day. I am encouraged to walk in the corridor several times a day. I have no pain, but am so weak and breathless that 'walk' is a euphemistic term for what I am able to do. Rather do I amble; a kind of optimistic, soft-slippered shuffle that fools nobody, least of all myself. Yet doctors and nurses keep telling me how well I look, how great I am to be walking so much. At first, feeling so zonked, I resent this, but knowing they mean well, say nothing. Then, imperceptibly, over a few days, a strange metamorphosis takes place. Psychologically, I begin to feel a little confidence again, for the first time in many weeks, though in reality I am physically still very weak. Brian Maurer, rightly, senses this minimal upswing in my mood and fuels it further by telling me: "We are letting you home on Saturday. You are reasonably stable now. Your new medication seems to be working well. Your name is on the list for transplantation and as you live so near the hospital in case of emergency, I think it would do you some good to go home." He stresses that, at the slightest hint of chest pain, or even discomfort, I should come back to Cardiac Care.

□□□

St. Valentine's Eve. Early afternoon and I am going home. A cloudless sky, warm sunshine. After six weeks of the rarefied reality of life in the Coronary Care Unit of St. Vincent's Hospital, and the limited mobility forced on me by my condition, everything along the journey home seems unreal. The endless swish of traffic on Merrion Road, the speed dizzying after the relative slow-motion of movement in the hospital. The clatter of the DART train at Merrion Gates, crowded with people, goal-driven, huddled. My first glimpse of Dublin Bay: a full, blue and white tide, the red tower of the Poolbeg lighthouse stabbing the sky like a swollen, bloodstained finger. A giant freighter, high on the flood, jerkily edging into its berth behind the twin chimneys of the Pigeon House and the East Wall warehouses, like some one-dimensional cut-out, being levered into place as part of the setting for a mammoth stage production of *On The Waterfront*. And, distant, on its little tit of black rock at the Nose of Howth Head, the granite tower of Baily shining in the slanting sun, the white-washed out-buildings dramatic as some Greek monastery across the great blue and white maw of water. As I watch it from the moving car it looks, at this remove, in time and in distance, unreal; a toy lighthouse on a toy rock, in another time, a happier time. But, I know it is not a toy. I know it is real, for I spent two years living and working there, Monday to Friday, writing the book, *Bright Light, White Water* (the story of Irish lighthouses and their people). Somewhere, inside that dim and distant white compound is the room where I lived and worked, with a lot of my accoutrements still in it; books, files, a radio, a portable typewriter, a wardrobe of clothes, a couple of bottles of wine. Things I did not have time to move back home before the heart attack hit me. Things I had thought, in the past month, never to see again. But now, pain-free, albeit weak, going home, the sight of the lighthouse raises my spirits, and I make a quiet resolve that, eventually, the transplant over, I will go back to Baily, climb the seventy-odd steps to the top of the tower again, and look westward as the sun drops behind the lovely-ugly, smog- besmirched city skyline.

Coming home! What a great excitement there is about stepping back into a house I thought I would never see again. The first thing I notice is the smell of home, so different from the clinical smell of the hospital ward. Someone has been baking; the unmistakable, pungent aroma of brown bread, soda bread and queen cakes. And someone has been cooking with garlic. These smells, never experienced in hospital, hang in the air like undeserved blessings. Then, there is the carpet underfoot, soft, warm, springy; a luxury after the cold, hard polished surfaces of the hospital. I go straight through to the kitchen and stand at the big window overlooking the long, split-level back garden, and beyond, over the tops of the houses, Dublin Bay. From this perspective Howth looks like an island, and the Baily lighthouse, more part of it, less detached, than it did from the coast road. I go out into the garden, half of it in shade now from the shadows thrown by the westering sun. On the shaded side the air is chill, but there is some warmth in the sunlit side, where my old Shetland collie, Pepe, is lying. He rises slowly to greet me as I approach. I am shocked to see how much he has deteriorated during the weeks I've been away. He wags his tail lethargically, and gives me one or two token sneezes of recognition. No barking, no running excitedly about as he used to do. His hind legs are stiff and unsteady, wracked with arthritis. But then, I am not exactly sprightly myself. I smile as I wonder if I seem changed to him. I shall never know.

The early dusk seeps, like some subtle smoke-screen, out of walls and trees and shrubs and grass, enveloping the garden. Daffodils, growing in profusion in a bank against the wall, glow in the half-light; every heavy-headed, golden, trumpeting bloom seeming to be lit from within.

After tea I go to my study and just sit there and look at the books on my shelves. For, among the things I most missed during the long weeks in hospital were my books. I am not one who, when a book has been read, puts it away and never reads it again. I go back to it over and over; each time getting a new perspective on what it is saying, extracting some new meaning, using it as an antidote to the poison of life, as a crutch to help me through crises. So, sitting here, looking at all those well-loved and much-used volumes, I remember the many times in hospital when, apropos of something that was happening to me at that moment, I would think: "Stevenson...or Eliot...or...Updike...or whoever...had something wise, or sad, or funny, to say about that in..." But, of course, the book wasn't there and I would spend hours trying to remember the particular passage. It stimulated and frustrated me, simultaneously.

My first night home. I am tired, having had more excitement and exercise in one afternoon and evening than I have had in my six weeks in hospital. I have climbed the stairs to my study, to the toilet, to my bedroom, several times. Something I would never have done in hospital. In bed, I lie awake and am afraid to sleep. Away from the safe, insulated, bandaged environment of Coronary Care, I feel great unease and apprehension. Lying in the dark I watch the hours pass on the illuminated clock-face, checking my pulse several times, and think of Scott Fitzgerald's frightening summation of fear, apprehension, worry, in the phrase: "In the real dark night of the soul it is always three o'clock in the morning." Surely, one of the most devastating things about chronic heart disease is the arbitrariness of the attacks and the great feeling of insecurity this engenders. There is the constant feeling that one is about to be ambushed. And if I do sleep tonight it will be metaphorically, if not literally, with one eye open. As if that would help. As if such vigilance would keep the cunning killer in my chest at bay and protect my friable defences.

St Valentine's Day. Incredibly the mid-morning sun is warm enough to sit in the garden for an hour-and-a-half. The old dog, Pepe, comes and lies by the side of my chair. He is content to sleep. I remember how, just a year ago, in this situation, he would pester me with an old, half-chewed tennis ball, racing across the lawn to retrieve it, returning it, dropping it at my feet and whining 'til I threw it again. Now, his heart is so weak he can just about walk. I sit in the shelter of the trees, full in the sun, and read and think and doze, by turns, as the whim takes me. The great joy for me here is that reading, or thinking, or dozing, I can feel the warm sun on my face, and the light, cool breeze brushing my skin and riffling my hair; can inhale deep draughts of clear, fresh air; can hear the ceaseless twittering of small birds in the bushes and the raucous cackling of the inevitable magpies, as they hop belligerently from branch to branch of the big ash tree, whose buds are black and tight still. Things one misses badly in hospital, where, if one opens a window to get some fresh air, there is usually an outcry from the majority of patients in the ward to close it again. In which case democracy always wins.

Sitting here in the sun, between dozes, I read some autobiographical sketches by John Updike. By some weird coincidence the section I'm into contains the following description of his mother's death: *"My mother died on October 10th, 1989, alone, in the house she wanted to be in, where she been born eighty-five years and four months before. She was dressed to drive her car to a garage in New Holland, first thing in the morning, and a heart attack felled her as she stood behind the kitchen sink..."* They are calling from the house to say lunch is ready. I go in, ambling slowly across the fresh spring grass, new-cut to honour my homecoming, mindful of this latest intimation of mortality.

St. Valentine's night. I leave the 'party' early, around ten o'clock, and go to bed. I feel a little discomfort, but put it down to indigestion. By midnight I recognise the symptoms of another anginal attack. Over the next two hours repeated application of my nitroglycerine spray does nothing to relieve the pain. Then I feel the insidious slow stain spreading in my chest. Not so much pain, as enormous pressure...spreading... spreading. Spreading slowly, inexorably, like ink spilled on a sheet of blotting paper. And with it the constriction in my throat and lower jaw, and the unbearable heaviness weighing down my shoulders, as if two invisible giant hands were determined to crush me. This has happened to me three times before now and my initial impulse on each occasion was to fight it. Now, I know that doesn't work. This is the unmistakable build up to a heart attack. I ask my wife to call the ambulance and, inside twenty minutes am on my way back to hospital, just thirty-six hours after I've been discharged.

This latest attack has been very severe. Two weeks later I am still in Intensive Care. I am stabilised now. There is no pain. Just the legacy of the attack; an enervating lassitude that makes the most minimal physical effort difficult. Even holding the pen and scrawling these words on the page demands enormous mental and physical effort. I comb my hair and am exhausted to the point where I need my oxygen mask for half-an-hour. I eat some soup and, after every third or fourth spoonful have to rest; the effort of lifting the spoon to my lips is too much. The large, hardback copy of *The Collected Letters of John Steinbeck* is too heavy to lift off my locker-top, so I settle for a paperback, *Selected*

Poems of Robert Frost. Reading one of the poems, 'On A Tree Fallen Across The Road', I feel that, even if God's sole reason for sending this latest attack was just to make me read that poem again, it was worthwhile.

Not though we have to seize earth by the pole
And, tired of aimless circling in one place,
Steer straight off after something into space.

After reading this poem I am so overcome with emotion that I weep. Looking out of my large, picture-window, I weep unashamedly for what seems a long time. I weep out of a mixture of helplessness, frustration and hope. Helplessness at my weak condition; frustration at not being able to do anything about it; and hope that somehow, against all the odds, I shall be well enough again, sometime, to 'steer straight off after something into space'. It is the quiet time, after lunch, before the visitors come, and weeping I fall asleep.

◻◻◻

I am awakened by the hubbub of visitors in the ward. The tears have dried around my eyes and the salt is still tacky on my skin. Though I am not expecting visitors this afternoon, I ask nurse to bring me some warm water to freshen up. She, without my saying anything, realises how difficult any physical effort is for me, and gently washes my face and dries it. I am so overcome by her thoughtfulness and gentleness and quiet concern that I can only hold her hand and whisper "Thanks!" To say more would be to risk more tears. She understands, and smiles, and leaves me with the curtain drawn against the babble of visitors' voices.

◻◻◻

There is something very special about March sunshine. Something special in the way it waxes and wanes so arbitrarily, as the docile flocks of woolly clouds are stampeded across the sky by the madcap spring wind. I have been allowed to sit out this morning for the first time in nearly four weeks. Almost imperceptibly my strength has been returning. I am still fragile, but not quite so weak. The spring sunshine, and reading that poem of Frost's the other day have conspired to lift me a little, accept the seriousness of my situation, even to hope a little. I have also been thinking a lot about the hazards of transplantation, what time I may have left, and about reconciliation. There is only one person with whom I need to be reconciled and I feel I must do something about it now. I feel so vulnerable, so at risk, so isolated by my condition, so marginalised, that I cannot conceive of going on, for even another day, without making some final attempt to bridge the chasm between us. So, I am seated here at my little table beside the window to write a letter to the erstwhile friend, 'R'. When last we met, over two years ago we parted acrimoniously. I feel it incumbent on me now to seek some sort of peace, and so I write to the effect that while I hope my friend is well, I have suffered some serious heart attacks since Christmas and have spent much time here in hospital. I tell how each successive attack leaves me weaker as I await a life-saving transplant operation. Unable to say how that will go, or even if it will come in time, I ask if we might effect a reconciliation, unconditional, forget all our past differences, not apportion blame for all the hurt we have caused each other, but rather, in this extremity, just make peace, be friends. I offer forgiveness and ask nothing but forgiveness and friendship in return. Our lives are all about crossing frontiers, I feel; the ultimate frontier being death. But that ultimate frontier, which I may soon have to cross, is not the most difficult. The most difficult frontier of all to cross is that of our differences with others, of our battles with ourselves. That crossing calls for charity, magnanimity, courage and not a little humility. My prayer as I write is that we can both dredge up, from some secret, holy place within our souls, these oh-so-necessary pre-requisites. Accepting that there is neither need, nor time, for meeting or any long drawn-out correspondence, I write in hope that my friend will be amenable to my suggestion, and will again be my friend, as I am theirs.

I know I shall find it difficult to sleep tonight. Not because I have pain, but because my mind is hyper-active. The medication trolley has been and gone. The lights are dimmed and I have saved my sleeping tablet for a little later. Right now I can only think of the letter I wrote this morning and had an orderly mail for me. I go over and over it in my head, worrying if I was concise enough, placatory enough. Worrying if I struck the correct note of sincerity, without seeming to be self-pitying. Trying to imagine how it might be received and what kind of reply I might get in due course. Eventually, I decide I have done all that it is possible to do, or say. It is said, and I must now wait. I take my sleeping tablet and ...

The cleaning ladies, early every morning, come with hoovers and polishers and dusters to keep the Coronary Care Unit so clinically clean. They are mostly good-humoured, always ready for a joke and a laugh. One or two are grumpy, not very talkative, not very given to chat or laughter. But the cleaning lady this morning does not fit into either group. She is certainly not grumpy; neither is she over-friendly. She speaks when I speak to her. She always asks how I am as she dusts around my bed and replaces the water carafe on my locker top. For weeks we had not exchanged more than a dozen words every morning. That is until this morning, when she saw, among the books on my locker, *The Collected Letters of Dylan Thomas*, a large book with a picture of Dylan on the cover. Tentatively, she touched the cover, smiled and said:

"Can I have a look?"

"Sure, go right ahead."

"I love him," she said, laying down her duster and taking up the book. "The poems are great, but I never read the letters."

"You like the poems?"

"Yeah. Especially that one that begins 'In the mustardseed sun...' and the one about his daughter... 'Never and never my girl...' Is that how it goes?"

She knew Dylan's poems indeed and, in the way two people with a mutual love for somebody will, we fell to talking about him. She had left school at the age of twelve, and was never a great reader, she said. "Just Dylan Thomas and Raymond Chandler and the Sunday newspapers."

I told her I had made three radio documentaries about Dylan. The last was just a few months ago when I went to Laugharne with Dylan's daughter, Aeron, to record a programme on location.

"That's the girl in the poem," my cleaning lady said, her eyes wide with excitement. "Oh, Mister Long, I didn't know you knew his family!"

"Just his daughter," I said. But that was enough for her to feel an affinity with me for life. And when I told her that one of Dylan's favourite writers had been Raymond Chandler she sat on my bed and gasped with surprise. But, her real joy came when I told her that I had known Raymond Chandler and had made a documentary about him also. It was as if I had made her a priceless gift. I offered her a loan of the *Collected Letters*. She accepted shyly and was gone before I could say another word. As I enter this in the journal I can see her, in the little kitchen across the corridor, perched on a high stool, reading; Dylan's book in one hand, her duster in the other, and a weather eye open for the Cleaning Supervisor. I must ask her sometime how she first came to Dylan. The genesis of things always fascinates me.

Talking with the cleaning lady this morning about Dylan Thomas has set the mood for the day. It's late afternoon now and I've spent the whole day dipping into Dylan's poems and letters and thinking about Swansea and Laugharne and the good friends I made there; Dylan's daughter, Aeron, Gilbert Bennett, Lorraine Scourfield and D. J. Thomas. So much pain and hospitalisation in the past three months have distorted everything. It all seems so far away now; so well-remembered, but so far away. Like something that happened in a dream, in another dimension; surrealistic. Sitting here, contemplating whether I have enough energy to walk to the toilet, it seems incredible to me that, just a few months ago, I had the energy to get on plane and train and coach and make the journey to Laugharne. And, that there, in that switchback town, beside the ebb-and-flow sea, at the end of Wales, I found the energy to climb the steep cliff-paths, walk on the sands at low-water and sit late into the night in Brown's Hotel talking, endlessly talking, and being talked to. It also seems impossible to me that I shall ever be well enough to do all that again. Make a return journey. But, remembering what Oscar Wilde said: "It is in the mind the poppy is red!", I cheer myself by reading Dylan's poem 'Should Lanterns Shine'.

The ball I threw while playing in the park
Has not yet reached the ground.

The early April sun is slanting on my window. While it may be still cold outside, the glass convects some heat from the sun. The combination of the heat, and reading Dylan, and my medication, which I have been advised may cause dreams, even hallucinations, all conspire to make me drowsy. I drift easily into sleep.

I am wakened by the arrival of the tea trolley. As I sit and eat my poached fish and sip tea, I remember the details of my dream. If you could call it a dream. It was more a reliving of one of those Swansea memories, almost exactly as it had happened.

I had attended some readings of Dylan's work in a school in Uplands, near Cwmdonkin Park, the park near which he had been raised and which had been his childhood playground. The park he had written about in the poem 'The Hunchback In The Park' and in 'Should Lanterns Shine'. Toward dusk I had taken a walk in the park. But, on that particular evening, in early October, the groves, as he described them in the poem, were not 'blue with sailors'. They were bandaged in a bruise-grey mist that had insidiously sidled in from the sea, obliterating the houses on the park's periphery. In my dream I stand in the fading light beside the now deserted swings. A short distance away, some children are playing croquet, mere silhouettes, slightly out of focus in the thickening mist, like figures in a magic lantern show. Their voices, though muffled by the mist, are quite clear. The croquet balls are not visible, but I know they are there, for, just once I hear the unmistakable click of the mallet, and the further click of two balls as they touch eerily in the encroaching gloom. At this moment, I am sure I also hear the ball thrown by Dylan in that long-ago childhood time swish unseen through the dying evening. And, though I listen for what seems an eternity, I never hear it land. And so for me it is still travelling through space, and will, thankfully and hopefully, never ever reach the ground. For that might dissipate the bruise-grey mist of memory and imagination, dispel that oh-so-necessary mystery.

Tonight I am allowed to go and watch television. It is important to me only because it means I am mobile; can walk along the corridor to the TV lounge; can sit with other patients and pretend, for a little while, I am normal again. The television itself doesn't interest me. Just as well, for among the ten people present there must be three different groups, each arguing very vociferously as to what it wants to watch. The very powerful, all-female 'Soaps Lobby' wins in the end and they watch 'EastEnders'. It is more fun watching the viewers, noting their reactions, eavesdropping on their 'asides' than watching the programme itself. But I soon tire of this and go out to walk, as I am now being encouraged to do, a few lengths of the corridor.

The corridor is very quiet tonight. The wards are quiet too. Unusually so for the Coronary Care Unit, where there is almost always an emergency. Most of the patients are reading, their separate reading lamps glowing like little islands of light in the semi-darkness of the wards. The monitors above the beds in the Intensive Care ward throb out their endless message; good news for some, bad news for others. The shuffle of my slippers is the only sound as I amble up and down, up and down. In the TV lounge one of the male 'lobbies' has won. They are watching a football match. The ladies have gone to bed. In one of the two little private rooms, called cubicles, the door is open. A woman patient is sitting in bed, reading. She looks up, smiles and raises her hand as I pass. I wave back. Next time round she motions to me to come in. We introduce ourselves and she invites me to sit down. She seems very agitated.

"Can you get the awful smell?" she asks disconcertingly.

"Yes. Yes, I can."

"Dear God! I told him not to leave that cat in here!"

The cat referred to was in a cat-cage under her bed and it had defecated, more than once from the look of the cage. The smell was atrocious. The man she had referred to was, it transpired, her son, who had taken a shine to a female patient in the next-door cubicle. Nearly all of his visiting time was now spent there and not with his mother. Tonight he had collected the family cat from the Veterinary College, where it had undergone surgery and, rather than leave it cooped-up in his car, had left it under his mother's bed. He was still visiting next door. Miraculously, no nurse or doctor had come by to discover the hissing feline under the bed. But night medication would be arriving soon, and then, quite literally, the cat would be out of the bag (or the cage) and the smell (or whatever) would hit the fan. I was dispatched, posthaste, to bring back the errant son and help get the cat out of the room. A delicate operation on so quiet a night. But, fortunately, the room was near the end of the corridor and riding-shotgun on the cat-in-cage, covered with a head scarf, was accomplished without anyone seeing us. The malodorous cloud permeated the corridor and the cubicle, giving great concern to the staff manning the medication trolley. But, of course, as so often in life, the truth was so outlandish that nobody thought of it. One nurse, who kept a cat herself, came close when she said: "Well, if I didn't know better, I'd say we had a cat in here!"

□□□

This morning is a big morning for me. I am allowed to walk as far as the little Oratory in the foyer, accompanied by a nurse. As we pass the cubicle from which I helped remove the cat-in-cage last night the occupant waves to me and says, "Good morning!" in such a friendly fashion that my nurse comments.

"Didn't know you knew each other so well."

"Actually, we don't, really. It's a long story and..."

"My God!" she interrupts, "what's that awful smell?"

And, sure enough, despite the early morning cleaning and polishing, the whiff of cat still hangs in the air, all the way to the foyer.

The little Oratory in St Vincent's Hospital is indeed an oasis of quiet and peace. The foyer outside the Oratory door is, for at least twelve hours a day, as busy and bustling and noisy as the Arrivals Terminal at Dublin Airport. Here, at the veritable crossroads of the whole hospital, they have two shops, a busy Accounts Office, an information desk, an admissions office, a bank cash machine, a change-dispensing machine, service elevators, and a large area with seats where very young children, not allowed into the wards, are accommodated. And there is the constant flux of visitors, nurses and doctors. But, beyond the heavy, polished oak door of the Oratory, is another world. A small, circular world of individual oak seats and *prie-dieus*, a carved granite altar, and an absence of the vulgar statuary and fussy fitments that so often debase such places, distracting the mind and inhibiting any meaningful thought, prayer, or meditation. Freshly cut flowers adorn the altar, glowing in the burnished light filtered through the stained-glass windows. A tiny lamp burns perpetually before the tabernacle. The soothing odour of flowers, old wood and wax polish permeates. The aura of peace and quiet saturating the place is tangible. All this helped by the fact that it is never crowded. I have never seen more than three or four people there at one time. The occasional visitor; but usually patients, in dressing gowns and slippers like myself, seeking some surcease from the monotony of life in the wards; needing a climate conducive to meditation and prayer. The only sounds I have ever heard here are an occasional, unbidden, heart-felt, heart-rending sigh and a muttered, sotto voce..."Jesus, mercy" or "Mary, help!" I have often wondered, sitting here, what fears and despairs and hopes are resumed in the accumulated thoughts and prayers and sighs of those who come here in any one day. People like myself awaiting life-saving surgery; others recovering; others with terminal illnesses. All forced by illness, of one kind or other, to the ultimate confrontation, the moment of truth, the coming face-to-face with God, and consequently with themselves.

Nurse comes for me and I reluctantly leave. As we go I look back at the exhortation above the entrance: "Be still and know that I am God."

It is now almost Easter and I should be well enough to go home for the holiday. I am on some trial medication which is keeping me stabilised and relatively pain free. Just the occasional anginal attack. More than the attack itself I dislike the treatment for it; the two quick sprays of nitroglycerine from the little red aerosol I carry always on my person. The side-effects: nausea and a splitting headache, and the awful aftertaste, lingering like a reminder of death on the palate.

Just now Brian Maurer has made his rounds and informed me that I have an appointment to see Maurice Neligan, at the Mater Hospital, after Easter. This is to discuss my transplant with him. Relatively speaking I have been feeling so well this past week that the business of transplant had become soft-focussed for me. This brings it into sharp-focus again. I pace the corridor after Dr Maurer has gone and think of many things that need to be taken care of. I go back to my bedside and make a 'To Do' list. One of the items is...'Ring my friend 'R'. — no reply yet to my conciliatory letter of two weeks ago.' I ring, with some apprehension, as we have not talked for such a long time. 'R' is formal, tetchy, merely saying: 'This is a most inconvenient time to talk. I'll be writing.' No more...I wait...

Home for Easter, but on a leash, with conditions attached! I am allowed out on Saturday, Sunday and Monday mornings at 9.30 a.m., and must return each evening before 8.30 p.m. I am still on trial medication and so there is a need for daily monitoring. The joy of the early mornings when I am collected and taken home. The feeling of anti-climax every evening when I have to return. Reminds me of those far-off days at boarding school: elation on going home for holidays, depression on going back. Still, I am resolved to enjoy the few days of freedom. Secretly, without admitting it to anyone else, though I am reluctant to return to hospital at the end of the day, I feel a certain relief that I am back in that bandaged, secure environment for the night, should I have another attack. This, I suppose, is the beginning of dependency on a hospital staff and regimen I have come to trust. In a strange, insidious way it is also the beginning of a necessary, benign institutionalisation.

Easter Monday. Clear, sunny and warm. To Powerscourt waterfall with my family. My grandchildren, aged six and one, are with us. With this life-threatening illness I feel a great need to be with very young children; a necessary, reassuring feeling of being part of a continuum. Watching John, aged six, wade barefoot in the stream below the waterfall, and his sister Laura attempt to eat daisies on the grassy bank, I realise that we never really die, but live on in those we love. This is a comforting thought. Then, on the way home, I think of the reverse side of that coin. Do we not also, contradictorily, pass on the seeds of death as well as the seeds of life? I can trace no single instance, in my paternal or maternal antecedents, of heart disease. If, as the experts tell me, and I believe them, it is hereditary, then how do they explain my condition? It must, they say, start somewhere in a blood-line. Unfortunately for me, and future generations of my family, it has, through some maverick gene, started with me. Maybe...

Just three days after my Easter break and Brian Maurer tells me I can go home. I am on heavy medication and, in so far as anything relating to heart disease can be forecast, should remain stable until I am called for my transplant. When that will be is something nobody can even guess. It is a matter of waiting and hoping. My meeting with Maurice Neligan stands for next week.

These first days at home are difficult days. I have to rationalise the whole business of waiting for my new heart. I've been stable now for a few weeks; very little pain, just the odd anginal attack. Also very little energy; just enough to take a short walk every day. Indeed, I would say that my energy diminishes every day. This is the myopathy at work; the heart muscle deteriorating, unable to pump. Consequently breathing has become a major problem. A constant shortness of breath now. And not just when I move, or exert myself, but when I am resting. Often, lying perfectly still in bed, quite literally 'searching' for the next breath, I feel I am going to suffocate. This is the most frightening symptom of all; worse even than the anginal pain. Lying in the dark, feeling that life is slowly slipping away, slipping out of my control; suspended somewhere between life and oblivion.

I have tried to establish some routine to my day. I try to write for an hour or two in between the necessary rest periods. This is difficult. The heavy medication has affected my concentration, and I often sit for twenty or thirty minutes at the keyboard without moving. I am happy when, at the end of the day, I have written 250 or 300 words. Then, I remember how, before I fell ill, my average daily output was around 2,000 words, and my happiness is tinged with sadness.

Some mail, addressed to me at the hospital, is forwarded to my home this morning. Two 'Get Well' cards, three postcards, a bouquet of Masses and a letter, at last, from the friend with whom I wish to be reconciled. Well, the envelope doesn't contain the hoped for 'personal' note, or the 'Get Well' card; indeed, it is not from my friend, but from a Solicitor acting on my friend's behalf. It is couched in the legal bafflespeak solicitors deploy. Its only message is a threat of legal action for harassment, if I attempt to make contact, by letter or by phone again. I sit in the sunshine in the garden and weep. Pepe, in the uncanny way dogs do, senses that something is wrong and comes and sits beside me and I feel his wet nose nuzzle comfortingly into my hand. Though I am disappointed, I do not weep for my disappointment. I weep that such obduracy, such intransigence, can exist; especially where once there purported to be such friendship.

I weep because my letter, offering unconditional reconciliation, has been treated in such heartless fashion. But, most of all I weep because I consider how very differently I believe I would have reacted if our positions had been reversed, and my friend had been in a life-threatening situation, similar to mine. And, I think, how little meaning the much-used term 'Christian' has for many in our society; how archaic, how debased it has become in the currency of a land of lobelias, tennis flannels, social clubs, poetry circles, credit cards, dinner parties and decent, Godless people.

The warm sun dries my tears and I go inside to freshen up and get ready for my appointment with Maurice Neligan at the Mater Hospital later this morning.

Maurice Neligan begins our meeting by telling me that, from all the information he has in my file, he would assess me as being a very suitable case for heart transplantation. Starting on that positive note immediately gives me great confidence in this man. He takes me through the various stages of the run-up to surgery and then through the surgery itself and the recovery. Then, he asks, "Any questions?"

"Only one. When can we start?"

"As soon as a heart is available. And that's something we can't forecast. Sometimes we get two or three donor hearts in a month. Sometimes we can go for two months without a single heart."

"Well, I hope it's not too long. This old heart must be near the end of its tether."

He looks again at my file and says, cheerfully, "Well you have some good things going for you. Your weight is just right. Around eighty kilos. And weight is important. The average heart we get is from a donor of about that weight. And your blood type is not one of the rare ones. So that enhances your prospects. Your general health is good. Then, your outlook is a very positive one, and, believe me, that's a great help to a surgeon." I am glad now that I have not asked him any of the obvious questions one might be expected to ask. Like, "What are my chances of success?" Have not asked, not because I do not want to know, but because I feel it is unfair to him to do so. How can he tell, really? Better get on with what has to be done. Better be positive, and trusting. Better abandon oneself to the undoubted expertise of people who know what they are about.

He goes on to talk about my getting a 'bleep' and being 'on call', but breaks off as he notices from my file that I have not yet had a dental check-up. That must be arranged right away. It is very important that my teeth are in good condition. Much of the danger of infection after transplant surgery can come from infected teeth and gums. He introduces me to his colleague, Freddie Wood, the only other cardiac surgeon in Ireland performing transplantation. On the day, or night, when the donor heart becomes available, the operation will be performed by whichever one is on call. He also introduces me to Michelle Kavanagh, the transplant nurse, who talks to my wife and myself at great length about the operation and the post-operative care; about the medication and its possible side-effects. We leave the Mater with no illusion about what lies ahead, no possible doubt about the terrible seriousness of the whole thing. But, the people we have talked to have also imbued us with a great feeling of hope and confidence that all will be well in the end.

I go away from this meeting, this briefing, with a definite feeling that I have crossed the Rubicon, have committed myself to a procedure that will inexorably lead to the operating theatre and a new heart...and, hopefully a new life. Oh, I know I decided many weeks ago, when Brian Maurer spelled out the alternative for me; decided quickly, without any prevarication. And, I know, that up to the moment of going into theatre, I have the right to change my mind, to veto the whole thing. And, sometimes, during the past few weeks, when I enjoyed a brief, pain-free spell, I was lulled by some feeling of relative well-being, and a seeming possibility that I might opt out of transplantation and stay with medication. But now, I have no doubts. Transplant surgery is inevitable. No matter how well I may feel in the weeks and months of waiting that lie ahead, there is no U-turning now. From now on, as never before, I shall be counting the days, the hours even, waiting for the new heart to be available.

The end of April. Days lengthening appreciably now. Warm enough to sit out for long spells, most days, and write in the garden. I am using a portable electric typewriter. Progress is still slow, but I have improved on my 300 words a day. I can now manage 500. When I get too tired to write I read for a while. Eventually I fall asleep. My breathing is still poor; walking difficult; but no major attack now for three weeks. The heavy medication is beginning to have certain side-effects and I find these very upsetting. An occasional feeling of nausea, and a total lack of taste. Everything, but everything, is tasteless. A helping of the hottest curried beef, a bowl of custard, a lobster salad, all the same, all tasteless, all leaving a revolting aftertaste as if one had eaten old army socks. So this is part of what Brian Maurer meant when he said the quality of my life would deteriorate. I pray now, every day, that the donor heart will be available soon. For the first time the stress of waiting is beginning to affect me, and my family. Just in little ways; little tensions making themselves manifest in relationships; tolerance of each other's faults and foibles a little lower than usual. For me, it is as if some invisible hand is turning a giant screw that slowly shrinks my world, hair's-breath by imperceptible hair's-breath. The little round of my days gets ever shorter, ever more narrow; from one day to the next I become less capable of functioning usefully. Little things it was possible to do yesterday, like walking to the newsagent's for the paper, I find myself incapable of doing today. And, tomorrow? Who knows! Perhaps tomorrow I shall be incapable of sitting here and writing at all. My confidence is being slowly eroded. Though not my hope. My hope is, thank God, indestructible, like Emily Dickinson's:

> *"Hope" is the thing with feathers-*
>
> *That perches in the soul-*
>
> *And sings the tune without the words-*
>
> *And never stops - at all-*

This afternoon someone rang to enquire about me, and to say that a friend of his had undergone heart transplantation recently. He is doing fine. No problems. But, he had a ten-month wait for the donor heart. I doubt very much if I have that much time.

A night of gale-force wind and driving rain. This morning the storm has passed, skies are cloudless, the May air heavy and windless. The great bank of flamboyant daffodils, so lustrous and upright yesterday, has been decimated in the night. The blooms are dying now, lustreless, faded, prostrated by the wind and rain; a tattered, tangled mass. The first sadness of summer, to see these once lovely, luminous, golden blooms fade. Everything reminds one of the inevitability of mortality. Everything dies that it may live again. The continuum, the never-ending cycle. So, in reality, nothing dies.

Tonight I went out with my wife and daughter to celebrate. A triple celebration; they both share the same birthday and we have carried over my birthday from the end of April. My first time to eat out in many months. Allowing for the fact that my taste is gone, I still enjoy myself. You see, over the past few weeks, while I cannot taste anything, I have developed a very acute palate for the texture of different foods. So, making the best of the faculties I have, I enjoy a good evening. Toward the end of the meal I feel a bit tired, a bit stressed; feel the first twinges of an anginal attack. I excuse myself, go to the toilet and take two shots of my nitroglycerine spray. It works quickly. They suspect nothing and we are home before the headache strikes.

The headache, the hang-over from the nitroglycerine keeps me awake for several hours. I think of how adept I have become at covering up these little attacks, so saving my family extra worry and stress. I have perfected the business of self-diagnosis, or to be honest and call it by its proper name, self-delusion. I tell myself that I can judge, very often to a hair's-breath, how long I can stand the pain without crying "Help!" When the anginal pain starts I often leave the room and quietly take my shots of spray, and go back and sit with my family and wait for the pain to ease. So far, it always has eased. But what if a time comes when it doesn't and I start building to a heart attack. It may be too late to cry "Help!" then. At such moments I think of a small toy, clockwork car in vogue when I was a child. It had something in its mechanism which, when wound up and placed at the centre of a table, allowed it to teeter on the edge before pulling back to safety. I remind myself of this toy car. Still, in sleepless, self-searching moments like now, I perceive that what is ostensibly a considerate motive is really a selfish one. I must not continue to do this. It is not fair to my family.

Very early morning. I am up before anyone else in the house. Not much sleep last night. No pain, but I am restive, apprehensive. Bad nausea. I drink some hot milk. From the kitchen window I watch the mist come down on the Hill Of Howth across the bay. The white, terraced villas seem to tip-toe down to the water's edge; at this remove, like toy houses set on a toy hill; a kind of Lego-land. The fog settles, like a giant grey octopus; slow-moving, murky tentacles obliterating everything, blacking out the powerful beam from the lighthouse tower. It comes down to sea level, rolling like big puffs of smoke across the water. The boisterous, diaphonic foghorn on the Baily lighthouse reverberates like the bellow of a wounded bull. In a matter of minutes, as I watch, the whole bay area is fogbound. The end of our garden is no longer bounded by neatly trimmed evergreen bushes, but by a dense, swirling grey wall of mist. I listen. The normal stillness of early morning is exaggerated by the fog, bandaged by it. I am the only person awake in the sleeping house, perhaps in the whole suburban sprawl, perhaps in the whole world. I feel so alone, so marginalised. My apprehension grows with every monotonous boom of the fog-signal.

Lunchtime. The fog has cleared, but my nausea and foreboding have not. Unwisely, I keep a brave face on things and when the anginal pain starts I go away quietly and take my spray. But this time it doesn't work. The pain, the discomfort, grows and I know now that I am headed for another heart attack. It is time to go back to hospital. My wife is out shopping and has taken the car. My son does what he thinks best and gets a neighbour to drive me to St Vincent's, only fifteen minutes down the road. I am in such a state of pain and agitation and near-panic that I do not, as I should, insist he call the Cardiac ambulance. The short journey by car seems interminable. I am, quite literally, holding on all the way. On two occasions, as we stop at traffic lights, I feel I am about to pass out. Everything along the route seems unreal; the traffic, the people coming and going about their lawful occasions, seem part of some surrealistic dream. The only reality is this growing pain, this insidious tightness spreading in my chest; this constriction of my lower jaw, and the frightening gasping for breath. Somewhere along the way I think, "This could be it," and I wonder if I am ready to die. But, even now, in this extremity, my sense of humour doesn't entirely desert me. "It's too late now to make bargains with God," I think, as I brace myself to ride the next wave of pain. Once at the Hospital everything happens very quickly when you are a regular patient in Coronary Care and on the list for transplant. Within minutes I am rushed through Admissions to the Intensive Care Unit. Back again in a world of monitors, oxygen masks, drips and constant attention from doctors and nurses. The morphine works wonders in killing the pain and that, together with the other medication, contains the attack. Soon, I pass into a deep sleep.

Each attack takes longer to recover from now. Each attack erodes appreciably the diminishing strength in the old heart. Each attack also erodes my confidence, makes me feel like a recidivist prisoner, having to return again and again to hospital. Hospital which, itself, has become a kind of prison. From hour to hour now I live in constant fear; like a man playing Russian roulette, wondering which will come first, the fatal heart attack or the donor heart.

Three days after the attack I am just beginning to recover, but will be confined to bed for another week or ten days. My strength, and my morale at a low ebb this morning. I am reading 'The Irish Times' when

Brian Maurer makes his rounds. He asks how I am feeling. My reply surprises him. I say: "Brian, I'm feeling so awful that I've just been reading the death notices to make sure I'm still alive!" We laugh together, but know the situation is serious. Time is beginning to run out.

◻◻◻

Mid-May. The trees outside my hospital window are in full foliage now. Lying here day after day they have become a large part of my shrinking world; the trees and the copse and the surrounding lawn and the ever-changing skies. This is my world now. This scene framed by my hospital window. Watching the trees from early morning until nurse pulls down the blinds at night I can read them like a map, or a storyboard. I often think of them as 'time-share apartments', the various feathered tenants coming and going through the day. In early morning blackbirds and thrushes inhabit them, often waking me with their incredibly intricate arabesques of song. By mid-morning, though I rarely see them leave, the blackbirds and thrushes have gone and are replaced by the raucous magpies, swooping and squabbling, strutting on the lawn, hanging like tatterdemalion black and white flags from the trees. And, in the early afternoon a great peace descends. The magpies are gone. The trees are alive with smaller birds, robins, wrens, finches, twittering the afternoon away. Around tea-time the pigeons arrive, grumbling and rumbling like rotund, feathered barrel-organs. Then toward dusk the crows fly home for the night, taking forever to settle into the trees; cackling, complaining, squabbling, eventually settling. I can often hear them out there, long after the blinds have been pulled. Sometimes, strays sea gulls peck about the lawn or roost in the trees, their tentative, plaintive calling to each other reminding me of all the lonely cliffs and beaches I have ever walked on.

And, I often wonder where all these birds go when they leave my grove of trees. To what other groves, what other fields, what wild and windy pastures under a wide sky. And, rather than envy them their freedom, their mobility, rather than lie here and feel sorry for myself, I go with them. For, if there is one thing, above all else, this illness has forced me to do, it is to inhabit the kingdom of my imagination, enter it fully, take possession of it once and for all. For me, now, after months of shuttling between home and hospital, reality has become a very relative term. A year ago, reality was the busy life I had made for myself as a writer, broadcaster and lecturer. Reality was trying to find time for some social life, with family and friends in the exciting daily flux.

Reality was the odd game of golf, the occasional dinner in a good restaurant. Now, reality is something very different. Now, reality is pain and very limited mobility. Pain of one kind or other. The physical pain of my condition and the consequent mental pain of worrying about the well-being, present and future, of those I love. So it has become necessary to live largely in this magical kingdom of the imagination.

The May sun is warm. I have recovered reasonably well and am allowed out of bed this morning. Nurse suggests that Matthew, the orderly, put a chair for me on the balcony outside the television lounge. I sit here in dressing gown, slippers and pyjamas and read in the sun. Occasionally, I doze and the book falls to the ground. It's a blessing to have discovered this balcony, to sit quietly and feel the sun and wind on my face; to listen to the 'time-share', feathered tenants coming and going in the trees.

An unexpected visitor this evening, of the kind that really lifts the spirit and brings back memories. A young doctor, new to the hospital, working in another Department, who has heard my name mentioned. He is a radio fan and seems to have listened to almost every radio programme I've made. He comes to introduce himself and say how much he has enjoyed listening over the years. He is a Power from Fenor, in County Waterford. I tell him that I also am from Fenor. He is pleasantly surprised. We talk about the old place and I have the temerity to ask him "Which Power?" he is. There are so many Powers in that part of the Deices that one always needs to know the 'nickname', in order to place the family. He laughs and says: "Well, did you ever hear of the Sunshine Powers?"

"Yes, of course."

"I'm one of them!"

"Old Pat Lar?"

"My great-grandfather."

"You know how you came to be called the Sunshine Powers?" I ask, tentatively.

"No."

And, as he seems like the kind of man who would enjoy the story, I tell him. Way back, near the turn of the century, his great-grandfather and my grandfather were contemporaries. There was then, as now, a proliferation of Powers in the parish, only differentiated by calling them the Pat Lar Powers or the Mick Tom Powers, or John Andy Powers. My grandfather, with a touch of the poet and a dash of mischievous humour, decided to coin suitable nicknames for the various families in the Power clan. Nicknames that never offended; indeed sometimes flattered. So, a Power who was obese, and constantly wishing for some miraculous weight reduction, was nicknamed 'Skinny'. And a Power who was constantly complaining, about weather and bad luck, was nicknamed 'Sunshine'.

My doctor friend is delighted with this story and promises to come back to see me again.

❏❏❏

Once the gates are opened on these childhood reminiscences I have learned to go with the flood; abandon myself, unashamedly, and let the great wash of memories engulf me. So, tonight I lie awake, long after lights are out, and the rest of the ward is sleeping, and think about my oldest friends, my dead friends. My best friends from that childhood time. My grandfather and his contemporary and boon companion, 'The Gusher' Power. The Gusher was the parish gravedigger. From them I learned, jointly and severally, so many useful, useless, never-to-be-forgotten things, in that remote, long-ago land between the mountains and the sea. Like, how to bait a fish-hook; how to 'blow' a bird's egg and 'string' it for my collector's box. How to worry crabs out of rock pools at low-water, knock barnacles off rocks, and 'lift' eels out of the mountain stream that flowed past our house. How to 'tickle' trout out of the Annestown River, after dark, with the aid of a powerful carbide lamp. How to cut plug tobacco that resembled bog-oak, and fill the bowl of a clay pipe. How to handle a ferret, plough a furrow with a pair of horses, and how to dig a grave. But, over and above all those things, they both taught me how to love words, and the magic of words, and what it was possible to do with words. For, though born in the middle of the last century, when formal education was scant, or non-existent, they had both been avid, if desultory, readers. Desultory because, in rural Ireland of that time, the peasant classes had very little choice in what books they read, or even when they read them. Books fell into their hands by accident. My grandfather, thatching a house for some well-to-do farmer, might mention that he liked to read, and be given a couple of books. Mostly Victorian novels, or the autobiographies of old soldiers who had served the Empire on foreign fields; or the memoirs of robust, jolly, fox-hunting squires. Once, he had been given a complete set of the Waverly novels of Sir Walter Scott, and, ever after, these had taken pride of place on the little three-tier bookcase beside the old man's bed. I remember, at a very early age, losing myself in that magical border country of *The Heart of Midlothian*, *Rob Roy*, *Red Gauntlet* and *The Lady of the Lake*.

The Gusher in his avocation of gravedigger, was quite friendly with a succession of priests in the parish. Through them he had, over the years, acquired a much more 'catholic' collection of books than did my grandfather. He visited our house several times a week and often took me a book, 'on loan'. And each time there would be a certain ceremony when he took one back and gave me another. We would discuss the one I had just read and he would advise me what to look for in the one I was about to read. In Canon Sheehan's novels it was, "the way he told the story". Though, The Gusher tended to prefer essays to fiction. So, mostly, I was given books by Stevenson, Chesterton, Gissing, Hazlitt and Lamb. They were, he explained, the experts at "turning a fine phrase", and if I ever wanted to learn how to use words, they were my "only men". The two old friends were great storytellers themselves, in the oral, *seanchaí* tradition, and would always weave into the telling a handful of fine phrases 'borrowed' unashamedly from their favourite authors. The incongruity between subject and 'imported' phrase never bothered them, nor their listeners, and still, in memory, doesn't bother me. Indeed it seemed to add a certain piquancy; what The Gusher called "a stimulating blend of the two cultures."

They were in their mid-eighties when they died, within a week of each other. My grandfather of pneumonia, in hospital. The Gusher dug his grave, and after the funeral, distraught and depressed, went on a four-day bender. On the morning of the fifth day, the postman, on his rounds, found him drowned in a bog-hole at the edge of the village. The coroner's verdict was 'death by misadventure'.

It is good to be reminded of these two old friends. Whenever I think of The Gusher I remember him reading from an essay of George Gissing that began: "Fog from the Channel and raining scud and the spume of mist rising on the hills, have kept me indoors all day ..." And now, across the miles and the years, I can still hear the tremulous voice, the reverential tone of the old gravedigger telling me: "Sure, 'tis hard to beat Gissing for the fine turn of phrase." And, in that most secret holy of holies, that special country of memory and imagination, where best friends, like old soldiers never die, I answer him from my bedimmed hospital bed: "How right you were, Gusher! How right you were!"

Today, after last night's self-indulgent trip back to childhood, I have a great desire to read again the *Essays of George Gissing*. Resolve to ring home later this morning and ask my afternoon visitor to take in my copy. Though it must be six or seven years since I last read it, I can remember exactly which shelf it is on in my study. Later, looking at the stack of books I already have on my window sill and bedside locker, I decide against this. Staff are very tolerant with me. My corner of the ward is beginning to look like a small library and nobody makes any complaint. Indeed, some of the night-nurses regularly, when the ward is quiet and there are no emergencies, come and borrow a book to read. Robert Frost and Dylan Thomas are the favourites for this night-time reading. The current night-nurse is 'sharing' the book I am reading now, *The Songlines* by Bruce Chatwin. I have it all day till lights out, when she takes it, returning it every morning before she goes off duty.

The early June days are so sunny and warm, and I am, relatively speaking, so free of pain, that I can sit for long periods on the balcony and take the sun and the air. Incredibly, I am acquiring a good sun-tan! I am reading a lot, and writing too; keeping this journal and continuing with radio scripts.

Tonight, just after visitors have gone, another 'emergency'. Mind you, one should get used to 'emergencies' in a Coronary Care Unit, but one never does. The sudden running feet, voices calling instructions, as trollies and equipment are wheeled into place, curtains drawn, always surprise, always startle, always upset, always make one think... "Could be me next time!" Heart disease is the most arbitrary of diseases, striking as it so often does out of a clear sky, without warning. And, there is, invariably, so little time in which to resuscitate the sufferer. Seconds can make the difference between life and death. Only those who suffer from serious heart disease know what it is to live in the cloud of that constant insecurity. Only those who know the presence of the capricious killer in the chest can appreciate fully the hazard of living on the edge, of picking one's way, a tentative step at a time, through a minefield. With heart disease one is at hazard every moment of every day. As John Fowles says: "Wherever time passes, there is hazard. You may die before you turn the next page."

We listen to the frenzied activity behind the drawn curtains as the Cardiac team battles to save a life. One of the Chaplains comes and says the 'Prayers for the Sick'. The battle for the life goes on well into the night and is eventually won, or partly won; the patient is stable, but in coma, having suffered, concurrent with the massive coronary, a stroke. Wife, teenage children, other close family, take individual turns through the night, sitting at the bedside. Who knows how long or short their vigil will be; hours, days or maybe weeks. But, for the duration of it, they will camp, like some bedraggled, demoralised army, in the television lounge. In this extremity, when a life teeters on the brink, when loved ones live under the volcano, normal hospital protocol is suspended per diem, for the duration of the crisis. Next-of-kin, quite literally, camp out in the lounge, sleeping in large armchairs and wheel-chairs, subsisting on a diet of tea and toast from the Unit kitchen. Going out onto the little balcony to smoke a cigarette. Getting what little exercise they do by pacing the corridor. Walking as far as the Oratory. Never going far from the sick-bed, just in case ...

Today the necessary dental checks were carried out and I am well enough to go home again. Though, I must say, that each time I go home now it is with less excitement, less enthusiasm. I have such a record of recidivism that my confidence is low. It seems to me that I am merely going home to wait for the next attack. I try to fight this defeatist attitude, but am not very successful. I know how I feel, and I feel pretty lousy most of the time. Even at my best. My family try to buoy me up and are most supportive, but my insecurity and apprehension is communicated to them. Am going early next week to get my 'bleep'. Psychologically that helps; it seems a step nearer the new heart.

Walked with the old dog, Pepe, and my wife and grandson, on Dunlaoghaire pier this afternoon. Am very tired, and have had a great feeling of nausea all day. No anginal pain, though I do feel particularly apprehensive. The kind of feeling that I've grown to recognise so well. The kind of feeling that usually presages another attack.

The attack hits just as I am preparing to go to bed. It starts with pain in the chest, rapidly spreading down into the upper abdomen, not as it usually does upward into the neck and lower jaw. It is the most severe pain I've ever experienced. I use my nitroglycerine spray at regular short intervals, but it has no effect. The pain grows in intensity until I almost pass out. My wife calls the Cardiac ambulance and I am on my way back to St. Vincent's. A frightening feeling of *deja vu* about this. Another round in the endless game of Russian roulette. But, I am still ahead, still alive.

Though I am rushed through to Intensive Coronary Care, there is some doubt about this latest attack being a heart attack. It takes several tests and a scan to establish that I have a badly infected gall bladder. I should be transferred to the Surgical Ward, but the stress of the intense pain is so great there is a fear it may affect my very weak heart, so I am kept in Coronary Care. I have never experienced pain as bad as this. They control it well with morphine and I am on a no-solids diet for several days until the infection and inflammation begin to clear. All thought of the heart transplant must be shelved until I have the offending gall bladder removed; there is too great a danger of infection. And the bladder cannot be removed until the inflammation is totally cleared. Until then I remain in Coronary Care, with daily visits from the Surgical Registrar, who will finally decide when I am ready for surgery.

These last few days and nights have been like a bad dream. A dream full of monitors and drips and intravenous feeding. A dream full of vomiting and retching and diarrhoea and violent, disorientating headaches. A dream over which hangs the cloud of regular anginal attacks. There is much discussion as to which method should be deployed in removing the gall bladder; the keyhole method or the older method of lengthy incision. There is a fear that my heart may not be strong enough to withstand the longer period under anaesthesia required for the keyhole method. Brian Maurer consults with Maurice

Neligan and it is decided that there is a certain risk either way. So, it is left to the Consultant Anaesthetist at St Vincent's to decide.

The countdown to the gall bladder operation has started. I am transferred to the Surgical Ward on the top floor. I am lucky enough to get a window bed with a magnificent view, overlooking Elm Park golf course and away to the Dublin mountains. The infection has cleared and the drug Warfarin, used to thin the blood and prevent clotting, has been removed from my medication. It will take six to seven days for my blood to revert to its normal consistency and so avert the danger of bleeding. No pain, but very weak. My fellow patients here are a mixed lot, in terms of their ailments. Two of the five are here because of their attempted suicide; badly scarred physically and psychologically. One of them is given to quite violent spells and has to have a special male nurse sit at his bedside during the night. After two nights of this he is transferred to the Psychiatric Unit in another wing of the hospital. During his short, troubled stay he has upset everyone in the Ward. A great silence all day. I think a lot about him and try to piece together where he came from and where his future lies. So awful it doesn't bear thinking about.

A really warm, mid-summer night during which it was very difficult to sleep. Awake early, I sit up in bed and watch some of the very early players on the golf course; the real enthusiasts who start their round at 6.30 a.m. Several foursomes pass down the fairway past my window and on into the distance. Then a pair; a man and a woman. At first I think they are both playing from the same set of clubs, but discover they are not. He is playing, she is pulling his caddy car, but not playing. He is not very expert and, full in my view, removes a large divot, with an inept lunge at the ball. She runs ahead to collect the sod and replace it, pressing it into place with her shoe. Early morning togetherness!

After the early morning golfers have gone I feel a great sense of loneliness. My fellow-patients are still asleep; the ward is still quiet; nurse has not come yet with the early morning medication. I take up a book, Thoreau's *Walden*, and begin to thumb through it. I have read it many times and am looking for a particular passage, near the end, which I am sure will help lift me in my present mood. I find it, and read:

"I left the woods for as good a reason as I went there. Perhaps it seemed to me that I had several more lives to live, and could not spare any more time for that one. It is remarkable how easily and insensibly we fall into a particular route, and make a beaten track for ourselves. I had not lived there a week before my feet wore a path from my door to the pond-side; and though it is five or six years since I trod it, it is still quite distinct. It is true, I fear, that others may have fallen into it, and so helped keep it open. The surface of the earth is soft and impressible by the feet of men; and so with the paths which the mind travels. How worn and dusty then must be the highways of the world, how deep the ruts of tradition and conformity! I do not wish to take a cabin passage, but rather to go before the mast and on the deck of the world, for there I could best see the moonlight amid the mountains. I do not wish to go below now. I learned this, at least, by my experience; that if one advances confidently in the direction of his dreams, and endeavours to live the life which he has imagined, he will meet with a success unimagined in common hours. He will put some things behind, will pass an invisible boundary; new, universal, and more liberal laws will begin to establish themselves around and within him; or the old laws be expanded, and interpreted in his favour in a more liberal sense, and he will live with the license of a higher order of beings. In proportion as he simplifies his life, the laws of the universe will appear less complex, and solitude will not be solitude, nor poverty poverty, nor weakness weakness."

The summer dusk is so exquisitely warm, so tantalisingly oppressive. I lie beside my open window on top of the counterpane, my pyjama jacket open. From this Surgical Ward on the top floor I can see, between the trees, right across the southern suburbs to the mountains above Bohernabreena. The last of the westering sun has just left the higher peaks, and their outline is beginning to blur in a kind of theatrical afterglow, as if some lighting technician had got the 'mix' slightly wrong and, momentarily, given us too much gold. The villas in the terraced foothills are no longer etched sharp, gleaming white; they are blurred now, grey-white smudges against the darkening mountain. And, even as I watch, the gold is fading, and the great wide vault of the sky paling to milky white. I am for surgery in the morning. The offending gall-bladder. They've got the consistency of the blood right at last, but, with my heart so weak, the anaesthetic is still a major hazard. A consultant anaesthetist has just been to visit me. A fine man, in whom I am sure I can have total confidence, but not gifted with a 'bedside manner', not the best communicator. He is positively brusque in spelling out the risks involved for me in having a general anaesthetic. Now that he has gone I am in a state of great agitation. What if fate were to play the ultimate dirty trick on me? What, if, having survived the various heart attacks, I were to die under anaesthetic for a gall bladder operation? For the first time in my life I am filled with panic, real panic. For the first time in my life I am resigned to dying. More than that, worse than that, I am almost welcoming of the idea of dying; leaving all the pain and all the stress behind. Even though it is late, I take out pen and paper and begin to write letters; letters 'To be opened after I am dead.' I have finished the second of these and the feeling of panic is diminishing. I decide to think for a bit before writing any more. While thinking I fix up my walkman and play the wonderful music from the film *The Big Blue*. As so often in the past this music, given me by my daughter many weeks ago, calms me, makes me see things from a different perspective. I realise that writing such 'farewell' letters is very defeatist, and not at all in character for me. So I take the two letters I have written and tear them into small pieces and put them in my waste-bag. And, from that moment I begin to think positively about tomorrow's surgery. From that moment I begin to abandon myself to a Power greater than myself, to God, and leave it to Him to see me through. After all, He has a good track record with me; He's always seen me through, in many crises. I face into the dark now, filled with humility and hope, and a total lack of fear.

□□□

Mid-afternoon. Surgery over. Gall bladder successfully removed. Safe in my bed beside the window I float back to consciousness through the big seas of my anaesthetized dreams. For a while everything is distorted, visually and aurally. The images blurred at the edges, colours muted, slightly out of focus, but felicitously so, as in some Impressionist painting. The sounds muffled, as if heard from a great distance, like sounds bandaged by dense fog. Sunlight everywhere. As I struggle to get the trees outside my window in focus, lines from Merton's poem,

'The Storm at Night', come unbidden into my consciousness, and with parched lips I whisper them to the all enveloping, holy sunlight:

But see, how through the waterthrash of surf and reef

The mind fights homeward to the beach,

Works loose, half dead, from the huge seas...

The trees seem so close I might reach out and touch them. There is a cloudless blue sky and a sirocco blowing. The great wind boils in the tree-tops with a sound like surf pounding the seashore. The leaf-laden branches rock and creak in a kind of wild ecstasy that is a mixture of agony and exultation. The wind tugs at the trees as if it might lift them by the roots, as easily as it would stooks of corn, and fling them away. Incredibly, in spite of, or perhaps because, of my still befuddled mind, I have total recall of a moment when I was a boy of six or seven. I was walking with my grandfather under just such tossing trees. The wind was blowing me off my feet; I had to close my eyes against it, it blew so hard. I could hear the trees tossing overhead. I didn't like it at all and, as small children will, I grew very impatient with it and called out to my grandfather, "Why don't you take the trees away and then it won't wind!" I laugh now at my childish naivety, but think how natural a mistake it was to assume that by waving their giant arms about the sky the trees made the wind, rather than the converse.

A week after surgery and the wound has healed nicely. I shall go home next week and be fitted with my 'bleep' and start the, hopefully, not-too-long wait for my transplant. Mr Murphy, the surgeon who removed the gall bladder, visited me today. He is a man with a sense of the ridiculous. I think he really appreciated my response to his question, "How do you feel now?" "Great," I replied. "You did a great job. It was a good dress rehearsal for the real thing...the heart transplant."

Home now. Beautiful mid-summer weather. My stomach is very sore and I find it a great strain to walk. My old heart is fast running down and the anginal attacks come nearly every day now. So far, the nitroglycerine spray controls them. But I get weaker and weaker as the warm days and nights go by. And, a new development for me, I am finding it very difficult to concentrate on anything for longer than a few minutes. These journal entries become ever shorter. I read one or two pages of a book and then have to put it away. I sit in the garden, in the sun, but even thinking is beyond my almost non-existent capabilities now. I sit and fondle the old, sick dog, who sits at my side all the time and drift in and out of sleep, checking my 'bleep' endlessly, making sure it's functioning properly, waiting, waiting, waiting...

◻◻◻

Today a phone call from John McColgan, the independent film producer. He wants to come and see me about the possibility of making a documentary for television, a sort of 'video diary' about my transplant. I discuss it with my family. They think I should see him, see what exactly is involved.

◻◻◻

Deal done with John McColgan. He is to install a video camera, with microphone and monitor, in the house, and I am to record myself in different situations, and in varying moods, during this period of waiting for the donor heart. We have got permission from the Mater Hospital to film the actual operation and the recuperation. The whole to be edited, in due course, to make a sixty-minute TV documentary; a video diary. I am enthusiastic about this project, especially at this critical time of waiting, when I do not have the energy, mental or physical, to write more than a couple of lines at any one time. This new undertaking gives me a focus, keeps me mentally busy, and could be a great help to others in life-threatening situations. When one considers that every two out of three families in this country are, at some time, in some degree, affected by heart disease, the potential for such a film is tremendous.

◻◻◻

July. A veritable heat wave. My strength is so low that I can't even sit in the sun anymore. Have to stay in the shade and conserve whatever energy I have. The medication is keeping me reasonably stable and I've had no serious anginal attacks for some weeks now. But, the stress of waiting for the new heart is incredible. Every morning I think to myself, this will be the day. All day, every day, I wait for the 'bleep' to sound, but, so far, nothing.

52

Took the video camera, on its tripod, into the garden today and shot some good footage of the dog and myself. The garden full of colour just now. Great show of my favourite flower, sweet-pea. All those beautiful pastel shades. A bank of it eight feet high, and still climbing. Magnificent, delicate, subtle perfume; especially late at evening, after sundown, when it's watered.

Pepe very ill this morning. Hind quarters almost totally paralysed now and a lot of bleeding from the rectum. He has also lost huge quantities of hair from his back and is totally bald in places. Poor fellow looks like a clipped French poodle. The vet is helpful, as ever. Stops the bleeding, sedates him and gives a cream for the skin condition. But, the prognosis is not good. We will have to consider having him put down if his condition does not improve. At his age any improvement is a long shot.

We are into August now and the wait is really getting to us all. Physically I am not too bad, but psychologically I am very down. On a visit to see Brian Maurer in St Vincent's, he suggests a few days away for my wife and myself. No too far, in case of emergency, or call for the new heart. We decide on a farmhouse in County Wicklow, within the range of my 'bleep'. Just in case!

Leaving this morning for the farmhouse in Wicklow. I could not be more excited if I were going to Barbados. Yet another reminder of how relative everything is. After so many months in hospital, and so much time confined to the house, it is unfettered joy to be out in the countryside. A cloudless sky, with little cusps of early-morning mist still clinging, like tattered lace, to the edges of the woods. I feel better than I have felt for many weeks now, but perhaps that is psychological, rather than physical. Whichever, it is a fact, and I enjoy it for the moment. The one thing I can be sure of is that it will not last. All my experience of the past year tells me it can be, at best, just a temporary, brief remission. As we drive, I remember some lines from Emily Dickinson and, to the rhythmic hum of the tyres on the tarmac, I recite them aloud:

Exultation is the going
Of an inland soul to sea,
Past the houses - past the headlands -
Into deep Eternity -

Bred as we among the mountains,
Can the sailor understand
The divine intoxication
Of the first league out from land?

❏❏❏

We stop for lunch at a pub in the mountains, not too far from our destination. Great Hungarian goulash, complete with beautifully cooked red cabbage and a glass of red wine. Afterwards, at the Post Office, next door, I ask for directions to the farmhouse. The postmaster is an idiosyncratic little man. "Oh, you're goin' to stay with ma...ma...ma... Marcia," he stammers. But, I have a feeling the stammer is not a stammer. I have a feeling that he intended to say "mad Marcia", but in the interests of good public relations, thought twice about this.

❏❏❏

The house itself is delightful. A well-preserved old Georgian place on a wooded bluff, in a fold of fields, above a winding, tumbling river that sweeps into the near-by sea. Very well-kept, with exquisite period furniture. Because of my condition we have accommodation on the ground floor. There are strict house rules, enumerated for us by our hostess, Marcia, who, though certainly not mad, is eccentric. Her eccentricity is reflected in many of these rules. For instance, dinner is not served until 9.30 p.m.; breakfast never before 10.30 a.m. Both a bit late for the average guest, but I quickly discover that Marcia's guests are not ordinary, average people. They are mostly from mainland Europe: from Holland, Germany, Denmark, Sweden. The kind of people who love to find the 'hidden Ireland', as the tourism marketeers call it. A love of animals is fostered here. Guests are proudly shown the large dish outside the kitchen door, where a half-tame badger comes down at evening to eat the left-overs. And guests are introduced to the seven cats of the household, who glory in names such as Plurabelle, Anastasia, Ginnette, Napoleon. The idea of a Georgian farmhouse appealed to me when we decided to come here. Now, despite the lovely location and the beauty of the house, I am not sure. There is something twee about the place. And...the cats!

During the long wait for dinner we sit in our room and I am very tired and somewhat restive. This is the prelude to anginal pain and a great feeling of angst. A doubt now that the trip, short as it has been, is too much for me. But, I have, long since, got used to the idea of fighting the pain and the anxiety and the depression; keeping a brave face. This is just another battle. A phrase from an old musical comedy song, 'This is My Lovely Day', from the show *Bless The Bride*, always surfaces at times like this... *"And if our ship goes down, she will go with the flag still flying..."* I often think that, *in extremis*, we always have a choice; to stand up and fight, or to lie down and die. And, I'll be damned if I lie down and die...just yet!

We present ourselves for dinner at 9.30 p.m. The other guests are assembled also. We are to dine *en famille* at the big oval table in the dining-room.Outside it is still bright. The air is heavy with the scent of roses growing around the windows. Cattle low softly in a distant pasture. Dogs bark to each other across the hills. Cats wander at will through the lounge and dining room. It is all just as if it were carefully stage-managed for the visitors. Then, Marcia appears at ten minutes past ten, still dressed in her outlandish Bermuda shorts and T-shirt. She apologises for dinner not being ready yet. It will not be served until 10.30 p.m. There has been a *contretemps*. She has been very busy out in the farmyard. There is a cow calving. She hurries away to change for dinner.

After she has gone, a Danish lady, who has been here for the past ten days, is heard to sigh: "My God! Not again!This is three times this week this cow is coming with a calf!"

"But, how do you know it is the same cow?" I ask, in innocence and ignorance.

"Because, here they only have one cow. All the others are dry stocks!"

Touche!

Dinner, eventually served at 11.00 p.m., is a triumph, a veritable gourmet's delight, a feast. The camaraderie, the scintillating conversation, the good food and the wine, all conspire to lift my sagging spirits. They also conspire to take my thoughts away from the cats that roam the dining-room while we eat. I am aware of them as the brush my trouser leg several times. But, the *pièce de résistance* is the serving of the dessert. Marcia carries the bowl of trifle to the table with a large tortoiseshell cat draped over her shoulder.

"Speak to our guests, Napoleon," she encourages him.

We adjourn to our beds at 2 a.m. I am satiated by the fine food and drink, stimulated by the conversation and nauseated by the cats in the dining-room.

☐☐☐

I sleep well. Just now after breakfast I go to the kitchen to ask Marcia for a flask of tea to take with us on our drive. While she prepares it I watch as all seven cats eat scraps directly from the plates which have been taken from the table after breakfast, watching their long pink tongues licking round the edges. I find this revolting and begin to voice my feelings, but am cut short by Marcia.

"Aren't they great fellows. Cleaning the plates like that for Mammy!"

☐☐☐

Back in my room I hold a council-of-war with my wife. Though we have booked for three nights we decide to leave forthwith. I go to pay the bill for the meals and accommodation we've had, and break the bad news to Marcia.

"But you can't," she says, very affronted. "You've booked for three nights. You must pay me for that time. Anyway, why are you leaving?"

"Because of the cats," I say.

Touche encore!

☐☐☐

Back home, after this abortive attempt at a holiday break, I am going downhill rapidly. Anginal attacks are frequent now; kept in control only by use of the awful nitroglycerine spray. Nights are bad times, when, because of the extreme difficulty with my breathing, I am unable to sleep. So the days become long, arid stretches, when the late August heat and the sleeplessness of the nights combine to make me totally useless. My strength is at a low ebb and my concentration is gone. I write a dozen lines in this journal and I am exhausted, physically and mentally.

Trying to write a radio script this morning. Sitting at the keyboard I do not have the minimal energy required to hold my hands above it and touch the keys. I weep, openly. Weep for my lost strength, and for all the things I can no longer do. And of all things, not being able to write is worst. I turn to the video camera, with a tear-stained face, in desperation and shout: "Fuck! Fuck! Fuck it!"

September. Walking, or should I say shuffling, on Dunlaoghaire Pier with my wife and grandson and the poor arthritic dog, in beautiful autumn sunshine. A sorry sight we must be, the dog and I. Seems like only yesterday I went down to the lighthouse at the end of this very pier, with a camera crew from RTE, to film a piece about my lighthouse book. But, in reality, it was ten months ago. Seems like all that happened in another country of the mind, and heart, and spirit. A country to which I may never have access again.

The first of the autumn gales. I cannot sleep, so I get up and go down to the kitchen and make some tea and hot, buttered toast and listen to the wind from the north battering the house. It is three o'clock in the morning. All of this illness is not an accident. Of that I am convinced. Such things are part of a great design, a master plan. All of this illness is, I am sure, designed by God to test me, pass me through the fire, humble me, make me a better person. If I can survive it.

I finish my tea and toast and walk the length of the path that goes down the back garden. The night air is balmy, warm. The Baily lighthouse, across the bay, flashes its bright beam every fifteen seconds, totally dependable. A large ship, well-lit, moves slowly into port. A half-moon lights the garden and the bank of sweet-pea glows in the moonlight. The air is heavy with autumn odours. The sky is clear and the high wind polishes the bright September stars. I reach the end of the garden path and stand for a while and look out over the sea. I feel

I have come to the end of something tonight. Feel as if, from now on, in deadly earnest, it is truly a race against remaining time...

PART TWO:

The Awakening

The tongueless vigil, and all the pain.

A. C. Swinburne: 'The Hounds of Spring'

September and the days are shortening, almost imperceptibly. My old heart is running down, very perceptibly. Activity, for me, has to be kept to a minimum. My breathlessness is very bad and I need to spend long hours every afternoon resting in bed. I hate this. Feel a kind of guilt about going to bed in the afternoon. Feel I should be working. But I simply cannot. Most frustrating. I wait...

ппп

A September wedding. My son, Conor, is marrying Annette. I have been looking forward to this for many months. Now, on the day, it is a great effort to even be there. Bad anginal pain. I am reading one of the Lessons, and during the Mass have to use my nitroglycerine spray three times. Afterwards, at the hotel, I have to go to a bedroom and rest, before and after the reception.

ппп

The third Sunday in September. I have been feeling a little better today, for the first time in many weeks. I go for a short drive in the mountains and come back home for tea. After tea I feel like working a little at the word processor and maybe shooting some footage on the video camera. After all, I've talked to it in my down moods; why not talk to it when, relatively speaking, I'm not feeling too badly. I set things up and sit down to write. The phone rings. It is Lesley Costelloe, the Co-ordinator in the Transplant Unit at the Mater Hospital. They have a heart for me. Can I please be there as soon as possible. It is 6.30 p.m. now. Half-an-hour should do it. Not much cross-city traffic at this time on a Sunday evening.

Now, even though this is the news I have waited long months for, prayed for endlessly, dreamed of endlessly, when it comes it seems so arbitrary, so casual almost, that I am shocked. My initial reaction is to say, "Look I've just settled down to do some work. Can't we leave it for awhile?" But, of course I do not say this. Instead the plan we have put together many months ago comes into action. My bag has been packed for several weeks, in anticipation of this call, for time is of the essence now. I ring John McColgan, as arranged, and alert him to have a camera-man at the hospital. Inside ten minutes we are on our way; my wife driving. We are both remarkably calm. But, though I do not say it, I am thinking, as we drive across the half-deserted evening city, that this may be the last time I see all this. And so I try to see the best in the passing scene. But, hard as I try, it is difficult to find anything pleasing to the eye in the ugly incongruity of the development all along the coast road, from Dunlaoghaire, through Blackrock, Booterstown, Merrion, Sandymount and Ringsend. The extraordinarily tasteless juxtaposition of new blocks of high-rise flats and offices beside old period houses. The proliferation of plastic-fronted, garish petrol-filling stations and shops. I am sad. Are these the last images I am to carry into theatre with me? No. There are good moments too; the tide full, and blue, on Sandymount strand, so full it seems to wash the bright red tower of the Poolbeg light; the Baily lighthouse, white on its black rock, and far out to sea the gleaming tower of the Kish, reflecting the last of the pellucid evening light. A couple of old, rusty freighters leaving port and the Dunlaoghaire mail boat just left harbour and standing out to sea. My eye is like a selective camera, recording what is best, leaving what is worst; registering these memories I want to carry with me into... oblivion?

❑❑❑

John McColgan and the camera-man, Seamus Deasy, are waiting for us at the Mater Hospital when we arrive. They are ready to record everything from the moment of arrival right through admission, preparation and the actual surgery. Some of my family, and some of the Mater staff, are concerned that making this film may be too stressful for me. On the contrary, I find it stimulating and rewarding. Especially when I think of what such a film might achieve in terms of helping others like me to understand what is happening to them; help them accept it all, trust God, and the surgical team, and not be afraid. For, I am convinced, that fear and its concomitant evil, apathy, are the really great killers. Not cancer, nor heart disease, nor the hundred-and-one other ailments that plague our mortal state; but fear...fear...fear. So, it is good to be part of this television documentary, to be involved in it on this very personal basis. In a sense it forces me to look at myself in a very objective way. I am not really looking at 'myself' when we are filming. I am looking at somebody else; 'a man' who is having transplant surgery.

Any misgivings I may have at this eleventh hour, any vague, irresponsible, stupid, cowardly ideas of backing out of surgery are immediately dissipated by the reception I get at the Mater Hospital. Such is the kindly, warm, positive attitude of the nurses and doctors that my worst fears evaporate like early-morning mist in summer sunshine. It is like being placed on a conveyor belt, a conveyor belt of love and kindness, where every single operative's function is to relax me, envelop me in a cocoon of caring, where I feel totally safe. I am put to bed in a quiet corner of a quiet ward in the Coronary Care Unit. My family are made comfortable in a nearby waiting room. A nurse explains the procedure. Now that I am here and being prepared for surgery, there will still be some hours of waiting. Waiting to make sure that the available heart is absolutely right for me. If the heart is right then there is just a four hour time-frame in which the surgical team must work; four hours from taking the heart from the donor until it is transplanted to me. There is always a chance that, even now, at this late stage, the donor heart may not be just right, and I may have to return home again and wait some more. It is now 7.15 p.m. A doctor tells me that they should know, for certain, within the next three hours, whether transplantation goes ahead or not. They are hopeful it will, but cannot be absolutely sure just yet. The wait continues...

By 8.30 p.m all the necessary tests have been done and the orderly has come and shaved my chest. A nurse asks if I would like to see the Chaplain, Fr O'Brien. I say "Yes."

8.45 p.m. Fr O'Brien arrives and sits beside my bed. He asks me if I wish to make a confession. Again, I say, "Yes," adding with a laugh, "even though I have nothing to confess." So, we talk for a while. Talk about my long year of illness; how it has affected me and my family. And I tell him about the reconciliation I have tried to achieve with my erstwhile friend and of the totally dismissive response it has elicited. This upsets me and I begin to weep. I weep because I go into the unknown and unknowable with one slate left unwiped. I weep, not for myself, but for my unforgiving, intransigent, obdurate, and, it seems to me, selfish and faithless friend. Fr O'Brien opens his little silver vial of sweet-smelling unguent and gives me the blessing of the sick. He then goes out to talk with my family.

◻◻◻

After he has gone I am glad to be alone for a few minutes. Alone behind the friendly wall of the curtains round my bed. The ward is very quiet now. Most of the other patients are asleep. One is snoring mildly. A nurse looks in to make sure I am comfortable, smiles reassuringly, and leaves me again. I think of how every evil under the sun comes from one thing, and one thing only...selfishness. Every single manifestation of evil is born in selfishness of one kind or other. Particularly the insidious kind of selfishness that goes about disguised as something else, insisting always on its own way. Only one way to peel the lemon..."my" way! Or, the particular kind of selfishness that goes about disguised as integrity and honour and will not come even five percent of the way; the kind that screams "no compromise" and thinks itself virtuous and righteous in the extreme.

◻◻◻

10.30 p.m. A doctor comes to tell me that my transplant will go ahead. The harvested heart is right for me. I shall go to theatre around midnight.

"Do you feel you need a sedative, meantime. Something to help you relax?"

"No, thank you. I am quite relaxed as it is."

And so I am now. Just the news that they are going ahead is all I need. I ask nurse to call John McColgan and Seamus Deasy and suggest to them that we do a little filming. I want to record my feelings now, here on the verge of the unknown, so that others coming after me may have some hope. I surprise myself by being so calm. They had planned to give me a sedative, but have decided I do not need one.

◻◻◻

My family come in, one at a time to wish me well. First, my son Harry, cheerful as ever, telling me that Waterford have won their League of Ireland match this afternoon. Then Deirdre, my eldest child, so caring, so good to have left her husband and two small children, John and Laura, to keep this vigil through the long night. Then my wife, Peg, as calm and self-possessed as I am myself. When they have gone out I have some moments to myself. I talk to the camera. Talk about whatever comes into my mind. But mostly about the great relief it is to know for certain that the donor heart is right for me and the transplant is going ahead tonight. And I talk about how calm and relaxed I feel, how quietly confident that all will be well. It never really occurs to me that I may die in surgery. Such negative thoughts are for others, not for me. I am thinking positively right to the end. I remember that I owe my publisher Dermot Bolger a book, *Brief Encounters*; planned for Christmas publication but left half-finished when I fell ill. I think now, "I must come through, complete that manuscript."

I finish with the camera and am alone again. I think of Conor and Alison, my son and daughter, who both left for Greece only yesterday; Conor with his wife Annette on honeymoon, Alison on holiday. They will know nothing about all this happening until it is over. Right now, nearing midnight, they are probably finishing a meal somewhere or dancing in a disco. I miss them, but feel glad that they do not have to endure the long, lonely vigil of the others.

Midnight. My time is near now. My last thoughts are for my donor and my donor's family. While my family and I rejoice that the new heart is here, somewhere another family mourns a death that has made a new life for me possible. I weep, quite literally, for their loss and, through my tears, thank them for their magnanimity. I say a silent prayer for them, to the close and holy darkness, and also for my family and friends. With a special prayer for that irreconcilable, obdurate friend whose intransigence has caused me so much pain.

Just after midnight. On my way at last to theatre. Down the long, high-ceilinged, echoing corridors; past the sleeping wards, followed by my family. I wave to them as I enter the theatre, then the doors close. They go back to the waiting room to their long and tongueless vigil; I, to my pain. The pain of surgery; the pain of scalpel and surgical saw; the pain of probing, and cutting and stitching; the pain I will not feel, in my anaesthetized state, while it is all happening; the pain I will not feel until it is all over and if I have regained consciousness, try to move, or cough, or even laugh.

□□□

The next ten minutes are to be my last conscious ones for the next seven hours. I am prepared for anaesthetic. I have now entered a world of sterile chrome, steel and plastic, inhabited by green and blue and white-clad figures, all masked and wearing surgical gloves. The only features I can see are their eyes. They come and go with great speed, as distinct from hurry, their every movement economic and efficient. Everything about their demeanour bespeaks expertise, experience, confidence, and they fill me with confidence too. Their voices are soft, comforting, as they explain everything they do. Their hands strong, and sure, and gentle. Their eyes kindly, smiling, above the mask. Their touch is so deft that, before I am even aware I have had the first of the anaesthetic, I am drifting into...

□□□

During the seven hours of surgery I was, of course, incommunicado. Consequently, I take the following vignettes from my subsequent viewing of the video tape of the transplantation. It is not 'easy' viewing any surgical operation. This is particularly true when the patient on the table is oneself. But I had committed myself to making a television film about my transplant, in the hope it would inform and help those who might find themselves in a similar situation. There was also a lot of editing to be done. So it was a case of screwing my courage to the sticking point, buckling to, and getting on with the job. Those vignettes may not be 'easy' for you, the reader, either. But, as they brought me face to face with myself, in particular, and with the human condition in general, in a uplifting way, I believe they may repay the effort of reading them.

□□□

What a jolt to realise that the inert body, etherized on the operating theater table, is...myself! Myself, with unconscious eyes taped, chest open, the two sides of the rib cage held apart by sturdy surgical clamps. Myself, tubed with drips and drains, wired to several monitors. Myself, oblivious of the expert efforts of the surgical team as they labour, with enormous grace under intense pressure, to effect the transplantation of this young, healthy heart into the cavity from which they have just removed the old, exhausted one. Myself, the unworthy recipient of this most undeserved blessing; this gift of life, this 'miracle', this awakening.

Maurice Neligan is humming and singing as he performs this most delicate surgery. "I always hum and sing when things are going well," he once said to me, adding, "but when I reach a snag the singing stops!"

The singing stops at the point where they are ready to remove the old heart. Gives way to an exclamation, "Good God, look at this, we've got problems here!" There are old adhesions, from the time, nine years ago, when I had the quadruple by-pass. They have to be cut away and that is, to quote Maurice Neligan, "a slow, sticky business." But, it has to be done before they can proceed. It takes about one-and-a-half hours. Meantime the old heart is failing and ultimately arrests. Massage is futile and they can't get it working again. So, I am actually on a life-support machine for a time while they get the new heart ready for transplanting.

At this stage Maurice Neligan takes a coffee break and goes to the room where my family are waiting. He is extremely courteous and kind. Tells them exactly what is happening and assures them that, despite this snag, he is confident things will be all right. But, nobody can say for certain for another two or three hours. "We are," he tells them, "not out of the woods yet." The long, tongueless vigil continues for them; and for him, the battle to save my life.

The camera pans slowly over the operating theatre: the surgeons and the nurses in surgical garb, the anaesthetist and me. Me prostrate; me inert; me unconscious; me with the cavity in my open chest cleaned of all adhesions now, ready for the donor heart. And, the panning camera comes to rest on the entrance, through which two nurses wheel a small trolley with a blue rectangular box on top. The box resembles a hat-box, or a picnic-box, or a cosmetic wardrobe. The nurses carefully open the lid and lift out a bag filled with crushed ice. Through the sparkling, silvery ice can clearly be seen the bright-red, impressionistic outline of the 'new' heart; magnified, distorted by the ice around it, like some luminous, crimson sun, fallen from the sky into Arctic ice-flows. They lay the bag on a surgical table and begin to take out the heart...

For an instant the camera holds on the two hearts, the old and the new, side by side. It needs no expert eye, no medically trained eye, no special powers, to discern which is which. One is flaccid, shapeless, unhealthy, clearly dead; the other, firm, healthy, clearly alive.

The reverence, the gentleness, with which the donor heart is handled as it is put into place. Then the long process for the surgical team of making all the various 'connections.' Things must be normal, for Maurice Neligan has begun to hum and sing again. The surgical team are more relaxed now, they make little comments to each other as they work. Maurice Neligan turns to the camera and explains that the actual process of putting the new heart in place has been completed in just over three hours. That is great. Anything under the mandatory four hours is good. Three hours, excellent.

The donor heart is in place now, the final stitching being done. Maurice Neligan gives the instruction to remove the life-support machine and let this 'new' heart beat for the first time in me. It seems to tremble for an instant, then pulsate into life, beat after steady beat. And, as it does, two tiny jets of blood shoot up from the living organ. Instantly two hands come into view and expertly, adroitly, adjust some stitches. The little jets subside and are gone, the bleeding stopped, as if someone had used a touch of magic. My 'new' heart is in place, functioning perfectly now. The long night gives way to day. The tongueless vigil is at an end. The miracle, the awakening, is complete. It only remains to remove the clamps, and other paraphernalia, and bring the severed bones, the torn flesh, together again in a triumphant, harmonious, climax to what I see as a surgical symphony.

PART THREE:

Celebration

"Hope" is the thing with feathers-
That perches in the soul-
And sings the tune without the words-
And never stops - at all-

Emily Dickinson: 'Hope'

Waking, after surgery, in my sterile cubicle in the Isolation Unit, is no sudden happening. It is a slow, almost dreamlike process; surrealistic, ethereal. I have an aural awareness before any visual awareness. Sounds, tiny sounds, muffled, bandaged, very far away; like bells and voices heard across the mountains on a windless day. And then, ever so slowly, the first glimmering images, swimming into view, waxing and waning in a state of perpetual flux, before settling into recognisable shapes and order. A blue, gently rolling, undulating sea, tilting precariously from side to side, finally settles and comes into focus as the bed in which I am lying. A white leaning Tower of Pisa slowly materialises as my nurse. She leans, smiling, over my bed, to adjust one of the several drips and drains that anchor me to the various monitors. Countless refractive prisms, dazzlingly bright, swim all round me. They settle in time, and I see they are really the glass walls of the circular unit which contains me. Coming back to consciousness, after such a long time, and from such a long way off, my first perception is that I inhabit a space bubble.

My nose itches, but fumbling to scratch it, I am alarmed to find that I can't locate it. It is covered by some plastic object, which, of course I can't see. It is an oxygen mask and nurse, noticing my plight, lifts it for a moment, enabling me to scratch. That simple act is sheer joy.

◻◻◻

Now that I am conscious, my first thought is for my donor; the one who made this awakening possible; the one who has given me cause for perpetual celebration. The one, without whose generosity I would probably not be alive now. What better time to put something on video tape, my first impressions on waking with my 'new' heart.

67

□□□

An hour later John McColgan, gagged with a surgical mask, is here with camera and microphone. I am sitting upright in my very high bed, propped by pillows, talking to the camera, talking about what it feels like to have a 'new' heart. Both staff and John are surprised that I have the energy, and the enthusiasm, to do this. My own feeling is that, right from the start, it is better to take some little initiatives. It is going to be a long road back to full health. As the old Russian proverb says: "The journey of a thousand miles begins with a single step." This, then, is that single step, that first, tentative step. For, if I am not positive and, do not metaphorically speaking, get off my ass and do something, then the only alternative is apathy. And apathy is first cousin to depression, and depression is first cousin to despair. So, with enormous will-power and effort, I talk to the camera...

□□□

Many months ago, when I first knew I must have a heart transplant, I adopted many stances, deployed many little ruses to help me cope with the whole insuperable idea. One well-meaning, pragmatic, medical friend advised me not to think of the heart I was waiting for, the donor heart, as anything other than a 'spare part', so to speak. This proved to be, on the whole, good advice, and I constantly thought, over the long months of waiting, of my 'new' heart as a part of some marvellously efficient cardiac engineering process. I made believe that it was just a super-pump, ordered from a spare-parts catalogue by serial number, and waited for in silence, and in hope of early delivery. I am sure that, psychologically, it helped. But, now that the 'new' heart is safely transplanted to replace the old killer heart I lived with for so long, I am certain that I shall never feel like that about it again. Now that I can actually feel this donor heart throb and pump rhythmically inside me, giving back life where life had almost ebbed away, I am in no doubt that it is far more than just a 'spare part'. I am certain now that it is someone else's heart, part of someone else, someone's great gift to me. Someone who died, albeit not wittingly, or even willingly, that I may live. Surely then, it is incumbent on me to respect this magnanimous gift; cherish it, without cossetting it; treat it with more care than I did the old heart, while not forgetting that it must be worked always to its full potential. For, to me it seems, the heart is very like a thoroughbred racehorse. The racehorse is bred to race, is happiest when racing. So, the healthy heart is happiest when working to its fullest capacity. There are two kinds of healthy hearts: brave hearts and faint hearts. Brave hearts are positive, they push on endlessly, pumping, pumping, boats against the current of time, enhancing and ennobling the lives of those they touch. Faint hearts are negative, dithering, prevaricating, never stretching themselves, forever borne backward by the current of life, losing today the ground gained yesterday; forever seeking the doubtful security of the safety net. Well, to hell with the safety-net! Life is for living, life is for celebrating; particularly with a transplanted heart.

Lying here in my space bubble, after the camera has gone, I make plans for this new, strong, vigorous heart. I ask for pen and writing paper. Nurse explains to me that she thinks I have done enough for one day in talking to the camera. She is very firm; the whole point of being here in this Isolation Unit is to have total rest for a few days. As a special concession she allows me to have my walkman. I play the music from *The Big Blue*. It is magic. My thought processes, hyper-active since coming back to consciousness after surgery, slow down. The music relaxes me, calms me, leaves me drifting...

Two days after surgery and I am allowed my first visitors. They can only come in one at a time and for a short period. They all have to wear surgical masks. My wife, who is recovering from a bout of flu, is only allowed to come to the door of the unit. She stands there looking very forlorn and waves to me from the other side of the glass. Security is very tight in relation to anybody, or anything, from which I might pick up infection. Only the duty nurse is allowed in my space bubble with me. She is there all the time. When she goes for her coffee and tea breaks, or to the toilet, a replacement sits with me. I am never alone. Food and medication are all passed through a sliding glass panel in the wall of the unit. There is a constant traffic of nurses and doctors past my glass walls. Life goes on. I feel, sometimes, that I am living in a goldfish bowl.

The third day after surgery. The bad, hallucinatory dreams begin. Of course, I have been told, in the pre-surgery briefings, that this may occur. Even so, it takes me off-guard, in much the same way as the call for surgery did. Particularly as the first dream occurs, not at night, but in mid-morning. Not in the dark hours, when only the night-light glows in my little unit, and nurse sits quietly reading, and all the blinds on the outer windows are down, and the hospital is quiet, and all the traffic of white-coated figures has ceased. But in the middle of a bright and sunny morning, when nurse is busy preparing my next injection, and the only patch of sky I can see through the big, outside window, is clear blue, and the hospital is busy, noisy, and the traffic of doctors and nurses past my 'goldfish bowl' is unremitting; a blur of white coats and pale-blue surgical garb.

I am on very heavy medication in these early post-operative days, mainly because of the danger of infection and rejection. Consequently, I drift in and out of sleep a lot, right through the day and night. This morning after 'rounds' I fell into a deep sleep and experienced the first of these hallucinatory dreams. It started in a very innocuous way. I was travelling in an aeroplane when we sighted several flocks of what at first looked like birds flying on both sides of the plane. As they came closer we could see that they were not birds, but some kind of midget space-men, not more than eighteen or twenty inches long, and propelled by tiny rotary blades attached to their backs. At this point I wake from the dream, not to the reassuring comfort of my hospital bed and the serenity of my isolation unit, but to chaos. I am fully awake now, and the bird-men are invading the hospital. They have already come through the open, outer window, through which I could see the bright, blue sky, and are swarming all over the outside of my space bubble, their tiny, cloned faces grimacing, contorted in rage at not being able to gain access. Hallucinating as I was, I assumed nurse could see them too and shouted to her not to open the door. I knocked over the stand that held the bags of liquid for my drips. Nurse rang the buzzer for assistance and the incoming nurse did open the door, despite my shouting not to. The bird-men invade my unit and I have to be restrained from flailing at them with my arms. I am given a mild sedative, calm down and spend the rest of the day feeling very ashamed of my irrational behaviour.

There was a time last year when, hospitalised in St Vincent's, awaiting this transplant, I vacillated between the polarised concepts that every man is an island, and that no man is an island. Now, lying here with this 'new' healthy heart throbbing inside me, I know I shall never be in doubt again. How can I ever believe again, as I did for so much of my life, that every man is an island, when I carry inside me this heart, this vital, life-giving organ that once belonged to someone else? A gift that has come to me through the charity and magnanimity of someone I have never known, and will never know. Of course we are all part of each other, all "part of the main". But I smile as I consider the section of John Donne's *Meditation XVII* that says, "...each man's death diminishes me", and think how much a contradiction it is in relation to my heart transplant. Ironically, not alone did my donor's death not diminish me, rather did it give me new life, add to my stature.

September sunlight. Warm, golden, slanting through the big outside window and, quite literally, bouncing off the glass walls of my isolation unit. I lie here and think about the whole business of contradiction, and remember what Thomas Merton once said about it. I was spending a few days at Our Lady of Gethsemani Abbey in Kentucky. It was winter time. And Kentucky winters are cold and full of snow and searing winds that corrugate the snow, and drift it up against the knobs across the open country. Until the whole sweep of landscape looks like a desert of white sand-faults. A group of us had just come in from a walk in the snow, and were thawing out in front of the big open wood fire in the Guest House parlour. We were drinking tea, and had kicked off our boots and were slumped and warm, lapsed into a semi-somnolent state. We chatted easily, superficially, about which sign of the zodiac each of us had been born under. Merton, whose monastic name was Father Louis, came in and stood near us listening. Then, in that abrupt, almost dismissive way he had when he came across conversation that wasn't going anywhere, he said, very peremptorily: "Excuse me, gentlemen! Excuse me! ... see! You're all wrong. We weren't born under all those different signs... see! Taurus, and Pisces, and Virgo and whatever. We were all born under the same sign...see! The sign of contradiction. And that's important in life. For, it's out of that contradiction that we produce anything worthwhile. That's the charge that makes the spark that enables us to do wonderful things...see! That contradiction is what gives us the energy and the synergy to attempt all those wonderful, impossible things...see! I love to find that element of contradiction in people. It's so much more important than consistency. Consistency is boring...see!"

A great surprise this morning. A 'Get Well' telegram from Alison in Greece. I had thought we had ceased to have a telegram service years ago, but apparently only internally. I hope she is well and having a good holiday; not worrying too much about me.

□□□

My fifth day after surgery and all the effects of the anaesthetic have worn off now. My chest is very sore, not just skin-sore, superficially sore, but deep-in-the-bone sore, where the surgical saw has cut the sternum open; where the scalpel has wreaked necessary havoc on muscle and nerve and tendon. Under the dressing, that sits like a great, white toupee on my chest, I can feel the stiff, hard, sternal stitches, that feel as if they might, under any kind of duress, pop through the skin. I find myself thinking..."I hope they put everything back together properly in there!" And I laugh at my undeliberate, jocular effrontery. Nurse looks up from her reading and smiles and her eyes ask me what I am laughing about. I tell her. She laughs too, and says, "I hope they did! But we'd better not ask Mr Neligan!"

"No. He might not appreciate it!"

□□□

My sixth day after surgery. Maurice Neligan visits me this morning and a decision is made that I am well enough to leave the Isolation Unit and go to a cubicle in the Coronary Care Unit. Joy all round at this. Nurses, doctors and myself are all delighted. It means the first crucial stage of recovery has been satisfactorily negotiated. But, nobody, least of all myself, is in any doubt that there is still a long road ahead; a road strewn with snags and snares, and the volatile minefield of infection and rejection.

□□□

Nurse is listening while I ask Mr Neligan several questions about my surgery and my recovery. He answers me in great detail and very honestly. When he goes nurse sits on my bed and chats.

"It's good to hear you ask such questions," she says, "but then I suppose you need to know for the film you're making."

I look at her long, and earnestly, take her hand in mine and say, with great emotion, "I ask, really, because I need to know for *myself*. It's *my* heart, *my* body, *my* life, and I want to know what's happening to *me*."

"Ah! That's the best reason," she replies, not in the least nonplussed by my total, naked honesty. "Good to see patients who are inquisitive about their own condition. So many of them would prefer not to know."

After seven days in the Incubation Unit I am on my way to Annexe 2, the quiet little room tucked away at the back-end of the Coronary Care Unit, which has been home to many transplant patients before me, during their period of recovery and recuperation. I am glad to leave my space bubble. My days and nights there were not happy ones. Not because I didn't receive the kindest and best attention possible; not because I wasn't recovering according to schedule; not because my attitude wasn't right or positive enough. But, simply, because those first days and nights after surgery were disorientated times. My seven days in my space bubble were surreal. I am glad they are over.

Rolling down the long, echoing corridors on my way to Annexe 2. The high, beautifully vaulted ceilings, the lovely old woodwork on the doors and casement windows. This could be, design-wise, with its space and airiness, a hospital somewhere out of the France of World War I, or the period of the Raj in India. A poem in stone and wood.

Annexe 2. To be my home for four weeks. Four wonderful weeks when, despite one or two setbacks, I will make remarkable progress on the road to recovery. Annexe 2, where, in so far as one can say that one enjoyed being in hospital, I can. Annexe 2, where through good times and bad, I experienced more care, more kindness, and more love, in one month, than most people experience in a lifetime. Annexe 2. A kind of benign crucible into which I went timorously, my self-esteem and self-confidence sadly dented by all the many heart attacks, and ten months in hospital. And out of which I came, after much self-confrontation and soul-searching, a new man, with a new heart, and a new, positive approach to life. Annexe 2, where, during long days and nights, I learned that celebration has little to do with the externals — the parties, the drinks, the songs, the loud camaraderie, but more to do with the abyss opening up in my own soul. An abyss of silence and peace; a climate where self-confrontation and self-acceptance are not

just possible, but inevitable; the good, fecund soil of liberty and desire, from which all good things come.

Annexe 2 is a small room, about 25' by 11'. It has the same high ceiling as the corridors and one large old casement window. Though the window does not frame a view as bucolic as that framed by my window in St Vincent's, the vista has its own special beauty. City roofscapes stretch to the skyline, a south-east skyline, punctuated by old Georgian houses, a couple of church spires and, in the distance, the twin chimneys of the ESB power station at the Pigeon House. In certain light the chiaroscuro of slate-blue roofs, grey walls and old red-bricked fronts comes alive with a certain shabby splendour and would inspire Utrillo, that old French master who specialised in painting roofscapes. In other light, or rather lack of light, the whole scene seems washed in muddy grey, lustreless, lifeless, depressing; a challenge, even to the genius of Utrillo.

Directly outside my window, and a little below the level on my room, is a flat- roofed extension to part of the hospital. Ugly, concrete, covered with a couple of inches of blue-grey stone chippings. I am reminded of some lines from Patrick Kavanagh's poem 'The Hospital', written in another hospital in another time:

> *But nothing whatever is by love debarred,*
> *The common and banal her heat may know.*
> *The corridor led to a stairway and below*
> *Was the inexhaustible adventure of a gravelled yard.*

The essence of creating a climate conducive to recuperation is discipline and order. Of this I have no doubt. So many people come through surgery, but fail to make a full recovery because of apathy and boredom. And, there are few places more suitable breeding grounds for apathy and boredom than the recovery wards of hospitals. For having had the will and tenacity to survive the big seas of surgery and other crises, many patients founder in the quieter waters of the recovery wards. Having reached the point where they are well enough to be up and about, but not quite well enough to go home, they are like sailors who have survived shipwreck on a reef, only to founder in shallow water as they wade that last mile ashore. They wander about aimlessly, in dressing gown and slippers, bemoaning the fact that they have not yet learned how to 'kill the time!'

My first evening in my little room. I am still wired to several monitors and, for periods, on a drip. My visitors are now allowed to sit beside my bed, but must wear surgical masks and are encouraged to keep their visits short. Pride of place on my locker goes to the little soft toy, a white rhinoceros, given me by my daughter Alison many months ago, and my constant mascot in all my hospitalisation. I think a lot this evening, after my visitors are gone, about the business of 'killing time' and am reminded of Thoreau's statement, "As if one could kill time without injuring eternity!" I resolve, before going to sleep, to get myself organised tomorrow, even with the constraint of not yet being allowed out of bed.

□□□

In this annexe I am part of the general hospital 'routine'. I am wakened at 6.30 a.m. The night nurses wash me and 'make' my bed before going off duty. This is my first wakening in this room and from my bed I can see the sun come up over my Utrillo roofscape, the white dawn giving way to a great suffusion of peach-pink. The early-morning light tints every ugly component of the view with a hint of magic, softening the harsh black, brown, and grey outlines, as the sun clears the low mist over Dublin bay and the long, morning shadows begin to shorten. Breakfast is served between 7.30 to 7.45 a.m. So there, for a start, is an hour to utilise... As this first day progresses, I take pen and paper from my locker and make notes of how the day's events are timed; after breakfast, the gently tinkling bell that announces the arrival of Holy Communion; the rattle of the trolley with my morning medication; the cleaning ladies, working quietly, efficiently, but always chattering, always good for a wisecrack and a laugh; the shuffle of six or seven pairs of feet, as the 'team' makes its round; the consultant's visit, which can be something of a moveable feast; lunch; my own visitors; tea; evening medication; more visitors; lights out. Unused as I now am to any activity, the minimal concentration required to make my rough notes tires me somewhat. Not very much, but enough to make me sleepy. It gives me great pleasure to say to night nurse, when she offers me a sleeping pill, "No, thank you! I think I'll sleep alright tonight."

I ask nurse not to pull down the blind at night. Prefer to go to sleep watching the far-flung lights across the city. Darkness cloaks the sordidness of the scene and I can invest that darkness with any images I chose; the only limit, the limit of my own imagination. Tonight I lie, or rather sit, propped with pillows and watch a half-moon hang from the scaffolding on the steeple of the old church in Temple Street. The moon moves on up the sky, and the scaffolding merges into shadow, a dim outline against the lights behind it. The early October weather is still mild and the top of the window is open; a gentle, night-wind riffling the edge of the blind.

This morning, after breakfast, I am all set to take pen and paper and make myself a daily schedule. My plan has to be postponed. The transplant nurse, Michelle Kavanagh, comes and announces that today we'll have some practice in naming the various pills and capsules that comprise my medication programme. There are so many it is essential that I get to know them all, together with their separate functions, as I will have to 'manage' my own medication when I eventually go home. She comes to my bedside laden with boxes, bottles and a small, grey-covered book that resembles a prayer book. It is specially laid out, a page to a day, and is a log-book in which I must enter my daily medication. My first medication is due at 10 a.m., so we proceed with getting that ready, entering each separate item in the log-book as we go. In total there are fourteen items, made up of tablets and capsules. I select them from the various containers and Michelle double-checks them. This, she, stresses, must always be the drill; a staff nurse must always double-check. As I listen to her enumerate the medications, and their related functions, I think of Henry Reed's famous war poem, 'Naming of Parts', and smile to myself as I try to remember how it runs...

> *Today we have naming of parts. Yesterday,*
> *We had daily cleaning. And tomorrow morning,*
> *We shall have what to do after firing. But today,*
> *Today we have naming of parts...*

Shortly after she has gone it is 10 a.m., and I take my medication with a glass of milk. Holding the fourteen tablets and capsules in the palm of my hand, I look at them hard and long. Assorted shapes, colours and sizes, one of the steroids the biggest capsule I've ever seen, a real gob-stopper. Surely, one would think that, taking this fistful of medication, not just once, but twice a day, was tantamount to overdosing. Yet, I know it is all necessary, to counter rejection, and all the many forms of infection to which I am now so vulnerable.

Good news after lunch. The great wad of dressing on my chest is to come off. This means I shall be allowed out of bed for certain hours from tomorrow; encouraged to walk, have sessions on the exercise bike in the corner of the room, and take daily baths.

Just before my visitors come they take the dressing off. My chest looks like someone has been playing noughts and crosses on it. The great central scar and the cross stitches making a definite pattern, all etched in dried blood. Nurse, very gently, washes the blood away. The outline of the, not unattractive, pattern remains. The air is balm from the open window, the sunlight flooding the room. I leave my pyjama top unbuttoned, just for the sheer physical pleasure of feeling the air on my bare skin. I am fascinated by the pattern on my chest.

I give my visitors a list of books to bring me. There is ample space here, on the little shelf under the casement window, for them. I am hungry for books now, my books. And I only have one book with me, Chesterton's *Essays*. I decide to dip into this while waiting for my tea. It is a pocket edition, packed in my 'transplant' bag many weeks ago, together with a notebook and pen. Now, Chesterton is always a joy to read, for many reasons. The elegant, rousing style, the irrepressible, offbeat humour, the wide range of subjects. I can always be certain to find something in Chesterton that matches my mood, or touches on something that is happening right now in my life. This afternoon is no exception. I begin to read the essay 'On Lying In Bed': *"Lying in bed would be an altogether perfect and supreme experience if only one had a coloured pencil long enough to draw on the ceiling. This, however, is not generally a part of the domestic apparatus on the premises..."*

❏❏❏

I have just finished reading this when Betty from the kitchen brings me
my tea. We chat for a minute, as usual. Then she asks: "Anything else
you need, Bill?"

"Yes, please. There is."

"More bread? More jam?"

"No, not that. You can get it when you've finished teas."

"What?"

"A broom, with a very long handle, and a piece of black chalk
tied to the end."

"Merciful hour! What d'ye want that for?"

"To draw on the ceiling!"

She looks at me, askance for a moment, then pretends to take my
tray away.

"No tea for you. What you need is a strait-jacket, a wheel-chair,
and transferrin' to Saint Brendan's!"

❏❏❏

A visitor immediately after tea. My friend Lilian Roberts Finlay, the
novelist and short story writer. Lilian is the kindest, the wittiest, the
loveliest, most caring of people. Typical of her thoughtfulness and
generosity, she brings me a very special present. She has been thinking
a lot about what would cheer me most, boost me most. And, in her
wisdom, she has decided to buy six copies of my book, *Bright Light,
White Water,* to send to friends overseas. My 'present' is to be asked to
sign them! The most welcome present, the most original present I've
ever had. After all the trauma of the past year, all the illness, all the
hospitalisation, the disorientation, I am not quite sure who I am any
more. I feel I had a life once, back there, somewhere. A rich, full life,
of broadcasting, writing, lecturing...But so long ago, I can hardly
remember. Suddenly, this magnificent, thoughtful gesture reminds me
of who I really am. My name on the title page, my photograph on the
inside flap, the 'blurb' about me, all conspire to felicitously remind me
of my true identity. I am still alive!

We talk a lot, Lilian and I. Talk of what she is writing now and then
she turns the talk back to me.

"You poor, poor man. Your life has been so disrupted. You have suffered so much this past year. How can you, Bill, have all this...all this, awful thing happen to you...how can you go through all this and still believe in God?"

"Lilian, my dear friend, how could I have all this happen to me and *not* believe in God!"

◻◻◻

It is after midnight now and night nurse comes to check if I am asleep. She surprises me by telling me I have a visitor. My late caller is Eleanor who is to have heart transplantation tomorrow. She cannot sleep. She is worried about the surgery. Nurse thinks it might help if she talks me. We know each other from St Vincent's, where she too has been a recidivist patient of Brian Maurer's. She sits on the side of my bed and we talk for half-an-hour. She is obviously cheered by how well I look, so soon after surgery, how strong my voice is, how positive I am about recovery. Eleanor always had a great sense of humour, and as she leaves she turns to nurse.

"Whatever Bill's had, I want too!"

◻◻◻

I waken in the night. There is a high wind and rain against the window panes. I lie awake and think about Eleanor and her transplant looming close now. I whisper a quiet prayer for her, and for the donor, and the donor's family And also for Maurice Neligan, that God may keep his eyes sharp and his hands steady, and that, this time, his humming and singing in theatre may never stop!

◻◻◻

My priority this morning, now that I am over surgery and beginning to recover, is to take pen and paper and make myself a daily schedule. Rising at 6.30 a.m. is mandatory, so the day starts from there...

6.30 a.m. Rise. Wash and shave at the wash-basin in the corner of the room. My chest is so sore, the movement of my arms so restricted by muscular stiffness that nurse has to get my toilet bag and towel from my locker for me. I am too weak to stand while washing and shaving. I sit. Impossible to raise my right hand above shoulder level to comb my hair. But good to be self-sufficient enough to wash and shave without help, albeit very slowly. The whole, simple operation takes half-an-hour.

7.00 a.m. I sit, in dressing gown, pyjamas and slippers, in an armchair at the casement window. The early morning light is always wonderful, even when filtered through cloud and city smog. And, sometimes, on clear mornings, the sky to the east, behind the Pigeon House, is awash with colour; a vast gentleness of sky; all peach-pink with little drifting cusps of cloud. A good time this for some reflective, spiritual reading. I start today with Thomas Merton's *Asian Journal*, a veritable treasure house of Eastern wisdom and joy. Like this: *"Apart from the daily experience there is no religious life, so satori (awakening, enlightenment) is an occurrence of daily life with its joys and sorrows."* And this, about the real meaning of real love: *"True love requires contact with the truth, and the truth must be found in solitude. The ability to bear solitude, and to spend long stretches of time alone by oneself in quiet meditation, is therefore one of the more elementary qualifications for those who aspire towards selfless love."*

7.45 a.m. Breakfast. The food is very good in the Mater. Fresh grapefruit, porridge, brown bread. And I take milk, rather than tea, my stomach upset, as it is, by the heavy medication.

8.15 a.m. Sometime between now and 10.00 a.m., when I take my morning medication, the cardiac surgical team — surgeons, physicians, nurses — will make their rounds. And the cleaning ladies will come in and sweep and dust and polish. It is a good, quiet time in which to write. Especially before my medication. Because, for two hours or so after medication I suffer from double-vision and tremors in my hands. I start this morning by writing a radio talk. So used am I to working on a word-processor that, composing with pen and paper seems very cumbersome and slow. And my thought processes seem slower also. I persevere.

9.10 a.m. Maurice Neligan and team visit me. They're happy with my progress. My stitches can be taken out in a day or two and I am to start walking, as far as the corridor to begin with. And, after the stitches come out, I am to start on the exercise bike. This is cheering news. I celebrate with an extra glass of milk at tea break!

10.00 a.m. Medication. The ritualistic selecting and counting of tablet and capsule. Then, the careful entering in my 'log-book'. I wait for staff nurse to check them. Depressing! The newsvendor comes round. I take two papers every day: one Irish, one English.

10. 15 a.m. I can now write again for a while until the medication begins to have effect.

11.00 a.m. I lie on my bed and rest. Listen to some music. Watch my hands tremble, and my fingers go rigid with muscular spasm. Close my eyes tight when the double vision hits...All side-effects of the medication.

12.30 p.m. Lunch. The food is fine, but I don't enjoy it very much today. The medication is beginning to affect my palate. Very little sense of taste.

1.00 p.m. I get into bed and sleep for an hour.

2.00 p.m. I have an hour or more now before my visitors come, so I take out my writing board and start writing. I have a backlog of letters to write. Letters to people who have written wishing me well. Letters to friends. Letters to people who, until this crisis, I would have thought mere acquaintances. Letters to people I have never met, but who are regular listeners to my radio programmes. The orderly is very surprised when I give him twelve letters, all stamped and ready for mailing.

3.15 p.m. Visitors. Family, friends, acquaintances. I enjoy my visitors. Can never have too many, or too much, of them. Each one of them brings, in addition to his or her own personality, a slice-of-life into the bandaged, insulated world of my hospital room. A reminder of what life is like 'out there'; a life I've lost touch with during the past year.

5.00 p.m. Tea. Mostly, I enjoy tea. It's sufficiently distanced from my morning medication, and my visitors have usually stimulated me, made me feel 'normal' again, given me an appetite for food and life.

5.30 p.m. I listen to the radio or watch television. News and 'newsy' programmes. Keep myself informed about what is happening out there.

7.00 p.m. More visitors. Usually, just close family at night. They can linger a little longer at night; stay on a while after the bell has gone, especially as I am in an annexe on my own. More than afternoon visitors, I miss my night visitors when they have gone. I follow them, with my mind's eye, as they drive home through city streets and suburban roads...

9.00 p.m. I watch the 'News' on television. All politics and sport!

10.00 p.m. Get my night medication ready for nurse to check. Then the handful of tablets and capsules again. I have learned now that it is easier to swallow all fourteen together with some milk. I now get into bed and settle down. Listen to some music. Fall asleep before 10.30.

Have my stitches taken out this morning. Worried a bit about this. There were so many of them. It didn't hurt a bit. Nurse had a very gentle, caring touch and it was all over in ten to fifteen minutes. I am to take my first walk this afternoon. I ring John McColgan to arrange a cameraman. We want some shots for highlights of the recuperation for the TV documentary.

My first walk, just as far as the corridor. I put on a surgical mask to prevent any infection. Nurse holds my arm, at elbow and wrist. She is very shy of the camera tracking in front of us. I am nervous at every step. Great weakness in my knees; feeling as if my legs were about to buckle and collapse. My chest is still very sore. Every tentative step reflected in little jabs of pain in my sternum. We reach the door without mishap or undue difficulty; then back again. Tomorrow, we will go a little further and I am to have my first physiotherapy session on the exercise bike. I am very excited. This is real progress!

Last night I had an extraordinarily graphic, frightening, but ultimately funny, dream. In this dream I had now been in hospital for over ten weeks. I had made good progress on the road to recovery. There were no snags; yet, every time I enquired about going home I was fobbed off with "Very soon now", or "Doctor will talk to you about that". Even my wife was evasive and, in reply to my questions, kept referring me to hospital staff. I became more and more agitated, knowing I was well enough to be home. Then, one afternoon I discovered, quite by accident, why I was being kept in hospital. While walking in the corridor, I overheard a doctor on the telephone to my wife. He and she were working in collusion to keep me there. Apparently the doctor had discovered that the skin could be removed from my chest every night while I was sleeping and a new skin grown within hours before I woke. The pattern left by the scar and stitches reproduced itself on each new growth. And this pattern was the big attraction. The doctor had a friend in the leather-goods business and was selling him one of my patterned skins every day, and sharing the profits with my wife. The skins were being specially treated and made into very expensive 'fashion' handbags, with the 'pattern' showing on the front. I was preparing to take legal action to have myself discharged from hospital, and acquire some of the profits from this nefarious traffic in human skin, when I woke...

Camera in today to record my first session on the exercise bike. A great feeling of 'progression' ...from walking yesterday to exercise bike today. Physically and psychologically this is good for me. I like the rhythm of pedalling, even though I'm not going anywhere. A great feeling of well-being afterwards. Reminds me of my cycle-racing days, forty years ago. How fit I was then! A fifty- to sixty- mile training spin every night. Racing every week-end. National, provincial and county championship wins. Best of all I liked the grass-track races. It was the end of an era then — the 1950s. Grass-track cycle-racing was still popular, every sports meeting having its quota of cycle races in addition to track and field events. We used steel-rimmed wheels for road racing and cane-rimmed wheels for grass-track. I remember cycling over sixty miles on summer Sundays to sports meetings, my cane-rimmed wheels strapped to my back. After a short rest and a quick change of wheels I would ride four, sometimes five, races on the grass. Afterwards a meal in some small cafe and the long ride home again. When I first began to have heart trouble, I used to wonder if that strenuous work on the racing bike had affected my heart, all those years ago. Talked to several cardiologists about it, but all were certain it had not.

Every morning, since I've been in this room, before breakfast, a large grey and white brindled cat lopes slowly across the flat, gravel-topped roof outside my window. It pauses every now and then to sniff the air in an imperious way before sidling out of view between two tall chimneys. And, every evening, around tea-time, it makes the return journey across the tiles and shingles. Once, standing at the open window, I waved and called to it. It stopped for an instant, looked up at me, without surprise or fear, and then moved slowly on. For three successive days now it hasn't appeared. I have named it Moscow, after a cat I'd had as a child.

The cameraman comes every day now to record some aspect of my recovery, of my progress to wholeness again. This afternoon he recorded my first walk down the long corridor, down which I had travelled on the night of my surgery. I am now able to walk unaided, but with someone close beside me, in case I stumble or tire. Nurse sets my mark as the second large window from the annexe, about fifty feet away. I stop there, and sit on the little casement seat to rest for a minute before returning. For two weeks now I've been looking at the same scene, the Utrillo roofscape outside my room window, so it's good to view another scene. This corridor window looks onto what was once a very beautiful courtyard with a well-kept garden. But, the need for extra accommodation has meant erecting pre-fabricated units on the lawn. Sadly the garden element has all but totally disappeared; just an evergreen bush here and there and a patch or two of scrubby lawn. The buildings all round the courtyard are of the old, original hospital, cut-stone, beautiful. At an oblique angle I can just discern the end of the convent chapel, which I have been told is very beautiful and has a beautifully kept garden, out of my view on the other side. I resolve to walk as far as the chapel before too long. Ambition, like everything, is relative. And right now, looking out of this hospital window at this raped courtyard with its few stunted shrubs, it might be the Pacific ocean and I its only discoverer. I remember a fragment from Keat's sonnet, 'On First Looking Into Chapman's Homer'...

Then felt I like some watcher of the skies
When a new planet swims into his ken;
Or like stout Cortez, when with eagle eyes
He stared at the Pacific - and all his men
Looked at each other with a wild surmise -
Silent, upon a peak in Darien.

A wild surmise, indeed!

❏❏❏

Sunday morning. A quiet time in hospital. The camera comes in to film Maurice Neligan and myself in conversation; I sitting in bed, he seated in the corner beside me. We want to have a sequence in the film where those touched directly or indirectly by transplant surgery will have some of their unasked questions answered. We talk about many aspects of my long wait, my surgery and my current, good recovery. Then Maurice talks about the whole concept of heart transplant from its earliest days. I ask him if the operation has changed much over the years and he surprises me by saying it hasn't. Hasn't really changed at all, which, to his way of thinking, is a sign that it has always been a very good method of transplantation. But, he explains, the thing that has changed, drastically for the better, is the management of transplant patients after surgery. Especially in the area of medication. New drugs are constantly coming on stream and medication generally is being managed much more efficiently now than even ten years ago. More, much more, is known about infection and rejection, and how they can be countered.

Before we finish our piece for camera, Maurice and I talk about my future.

"You have a biopsy on Tuesday, Bill. After that, all things being equal, I see no reason why you shouldn't go home soon, perhaps next week-end."

"Great, that will be just about three weeks since surgery."

"What do you intend to do when you go home? And, I don't just mean in terms of diet, exercise, etc. I know you'll be responsible in that. I mean in terms of maybe a shift in life-style."

"Well, the first thing I am going to do is rationalise my workload."

"Yes, that's what I mean. How can you achieve that?"

"You know that, for several years now, I've been living three lives. Writing, broadcasting and lecturing, and conducting workshops in Maynooth and other places. Well, one of these will have to go."

"You mean, from now on you'll just live *two* lives!"

"Not really. You see the writing and broadcasting go very much together. There's a certain compatibility between the two. But, the lecturing. Well, that's very hard work. Stressful. Doesn't really complement the others. So I think that will have to go."

"Makes sense. I suppose moderation is the answer in all things. Even in moderation!"

After the camera has gone, Maurice Neligan and I sit and talk for a while. Before he goes he tells me how well I'm doing. Ethics forbid his talking in any detail about the donor heart I've received.

"You got a very sound, young heart, Bill. Should serve you well."

Later, I must have looked inordinately pleased as I told one of my visitors of my 'new', young heart. He admonished me, with a knowing smile: "Now, don't lose the run of yourself. Remember all your other organs are sixty-two years old!"

Sunday evening, when the last visitors have gone is a particularly lonely time in hospital. Well, every evening is, but there is something special about Sunday. And, it's not helped by the ennui that sets in after a surfeit of Sunday newspapers. A reading of every news story told with a different bias in each of several papers, each with its axe to grind. And endless opinion columns, agony aunt columns, and colour magazines where it's difficult to find the editorial content sandwiched between the glossy advertisements. I listen to *The Big Blue* and try to sleep.

I am wakened in the night by the wailing of an ambulance as it screams into the Casualty Department, just in the back of where I am. That sound is an unsettling sound and I can't seem to get back to sleep again. Night nurse brings me a cup of tea and sits and talks for a few minutes. When she goes I think about who might have been in that casualty ambulance. Then, I sleep.

A story on the inside pages of my morning paper. Headline reads ..." MAN DIES IN CITY STABBING...'A 29-year old man, of no fixed abode, died in a stabbing incident outside a city-centre public house last night. He was stabbed six times in the heart and four times in the upper abdomen and was admitted to the Mater Hospital. A team of surgeons worked for hours in an attempt to save his life. He died at 4.30 a.m...'

I think, sadly, of this wanton killing. Here in this very hospital where he died, there is so much time, expertise, loving care spent in saving lives, bringing them back from the edge, nursing them back to full health again. And this poor man is killed by a drunken whim, in a fit of passion, arbitrarily...Doesn't make sense.

The corridor is a busy place during visiting hours. Walking there tonight with my visitors, I experience the great joy and surprise of seeing Conor and his bride, Annette, coming toward us through the press of people. They are just back from honeymoon, tanned and happy, radiating the Hellenic sunshine and light in which they have been basking for the past two weeks. We have a joyful 're-union' right there in the corridor. Hard to imagine that the last time I saw them was on their wedding day just over two weeks ago, and that so much could happen, so quickly, for me, in that interim.

John, my six-year old grandson, came to visit me tonight and sat on the end of my bed and talked a blue streak for ten minutes. Told me all about his school and what he is learning. Also about what he's watching on television, and his swimming lessons. We recorded the conversation on camera for the documentary. He surprised me by not being in the least camera-conscious, but very composed, as if the camera were not there.

Result of biopsy this morning. I will not be going home as was expected. My rejection factor is a trifle high and must be brought down before I'm discharged. After some initial disappointment I am not worried about this. I am assured it is easily managed by a couple of hours on a drip every day for three days. After that, another biopsy, and, hopefully home.

I have built up quite a library of books and files on the shelf of my casement window. I was working there now, writing some radio pieces, when the 'team' made their rounds. The camera is now a permanent presence in my room as we are filming nearly every day. Some of the doctors express surprise that I am working so early.

"But this is not early," I say, with a smile.

"No? It's only 9.30."

"I've been writing since 8.00."

"Must be careful and not overdo things."

"No danger. Anyway, I think more people regress during recuperation from apathy and boredom than from overwork."

"Oh!"

I love that quiet time, after lunch, when the orderly comes to take me for my bath. The first few times I was very tentative in all my movements. Dead scared I might slip, or fall, getting in and out of the bath. But I've become more confident and enjoy the walk to the bathroom now and the bath itself.

Alison, just back from her holiday in Greece, comes to see me this evening. She is all bronzed and relaxed. Makes me dream of holidays in the sun. But, for the moment it can only be a dream. There is a way to go for me along this road to complete recovery before I start thinking of such things.

Another visitor tonight. A friend who has recently visited the Baily lighthouse. He told me, with great respect, that the keeper on duty had shown him my old 'rooms' where I had lived while writing the book. He described them to me, itemising some of the paraphernalia I had left behind. The keeper told him I would be back, after I had recovered, to write another book. What book? When?

Another visitor tonight.

The October sky is clear this afternoon and the light is good for filming out of doors. John McColgan has come and we have permission to go outside and film in the convent garden, and afterwards in the chapel. This is my first time to go outside since my surgery. I dress fully for the first time, but have to borrow John's leather jacket, as the air is autumn-chill. The convent garden is a little oasis of peace and love-liness; a place one would not expect to find in the midst of all these grey, towering buildings and prefabricated extensions. Outside the high boundary wall is the main bus-route to Phibsboro. I can hear the swish of the traffic and hear the distant screech of brakes, and see the bright green top of a No. 10 bus glide by. Thank God the nuns, in their wisdom, have kept this space intact. The lawn is lush and bright green, littered with russet-coloured leaves that rustle and 'walk' about in the light wind. Some pears have fallen from one of the trees and are startlingly yellow in the grass, where small birds hop and peck them. There is birdsong everywhere. In a pear tree, a song-drunk blackbird has gone mad, and somewhere close-by, a late, sun-drunk grasshopper, unaware that summer has passed, lisps in the long grass. I am tired after my walk from the hospital, so I sit on a bench in a sheltered corner. I am so intoxicated with this first excursion out-of-doors that I am quite speechless. I just sit back and watch, through the thinning foliage on the pear tree, the small islands of white cloud drifting in the azure sky. The warm sun and the thin, chill wind on my face, is like some divine cocktail. Instinctively I bend down, and cupping my hands together, fill them with fallen leaves. I close my eyes and bury my face in the leaves cupped in my hands, and hold it there for what seems a long time. I can feel the leaves crinkly and crisp against my skin and smell from them all the stored sunshine of the summer I have missed, and feel the refracted light of the countless suns and moons that have drenched this garden. Silently, I thank God for seeing me through all my adventures and misadventures of the heart. Thank Him for bringing me here to this garden to hear, and see, and smell all the beautiful things I thought I might never experience again. For, indeed, He has led me by a way I cannot possibly understand. But, then, it is not important that I understand it, only that I surrender to it, accept it as being the best way. He has brought me from the Munster glen where I was born, to Dublin, to London, to New York, to Central America, to Rome and back, full circle, to Dublin again, in order that I may come, this particular afternoon, to this particular garden, to give Him this particular thanks.

When John asks me to speak to the camera, I cannot. I am too emotional, too full of a mixture of joy and sadness to say anything. It will have to be a voice-over when we come to editing this part of the film.

The convent church is exquisitely designed, ornately furnished and beautifully, lovingly kept by the nuns. We film there for half-an-hour. It is some special Feast Day and the Blessed Sacrament is exposed, the high altar covered in flowers, candles burning, the flickering flames reflected in the shining brasswork. Several nuns keep vigil. Outside, dulled now by the thickness of the granite walls, the birds still sing in the little garden and the traffic is just a distant hum. I am a little tired now. A combination, I suppose, of the walking, the first fresh air for weeks, and the incredible feeling of knowing that the transplantation has worked, that I have a new heart and a new life.

Result of my latest biopsy is good. The rejection factor is under control, and I shall be discharged within the next few days. Rejoicing all round. I am surprised at how excited staff get about such things. Had thought that, because they have so many people to look after and worry about, an individual recovery would not excite them. But it does.

Into my room, this afternoon, came a man trailing clouds, if not of glory, then of Wicklow heather, mountain streams, peat fires, pine forests, fish and dogs. He is an old friend, a true eccentric and iconoclast; a painter from the wild Wicklow country south-west of Glendalough. He did not so much walk into my room, as materialise in the doorway, all fifteen stone of him. Clad in ancient tweeds, with the colourful flies from many fishing expeditions still stuck in his hat, and a purple weed tucked in his lapel, he ambled across the floor and besieged me with an enormous hug. He reeked of the acrid smell of peat fires, the homely odour of Wicklow collies, and the rancid pong of stale fish. Not one with much regard for personal hygiene, or, for that matter, hygiene of any kind, he nevertheless was a man with a soul and spirit big enough to have the virtues of his faults. He filled my little room with the very essence of Wicklow countryside; the high and open mountains, the streams in spate, the vast forests, the winding hill-roads. We talked for over an hour and when he got up to leave, he took the sprig of purple weed from his lapel and placed it on my locker.

"A wild-flower for you," he said, "I picked it at the roadside while waiting for the bus."

Then he was gone, ambling away as quietly as he had come, taking my thoughts and my heart with him to the mountain fastness where he lived with his dogs, and his fish, and his bright peat fires. And, long after he was gone, the bitter-sweet smell of peat smoke lingered in the clinical, sterile, hospital air.

At last. Going home. The excitement of packing all my clothes and books and various files and papers. The briefing from Michelle Kavanagh, the transplant nurse, who will, henceforth, be my point of contact with Coronary Care at the hospital. The reminders about my medication, the possible side-effects of that medication. Instructions about when to come for regular blood test and periodic biopsy. Directives about food; no pork, no shell fish, no lettuce, no vegetables or fruit with skins, no tap water, no full-fat milk, no non-pasteurised cheese. And very strict rules about hygiene; a bath every day, and hair-wash every day. No showers, as a lot of infection can come from the shower head. Stay clear of smokey, dust-laden environments. Above all, contact the hospital on the first manifestation of any infection, illness, soreness, pain. A warning that I may suffer some depression after I've left the hospital; may feel insecure.

The camera has come to record my going home and so I am disappointed that I have to leave the actual hospital in a wheel-chair. It is a strict rule that all transplant patients are wheeled to the waiting car. My goodbye to Michelle, who accompanied me to the car, is a tearful one. I am very emotional. She is emotional too. We both know how close I have come to the edge of life.

"Please go," she says, with mock gruffness, "before you have me crying too!"

◻◻◻

My first night home. No feelings yet of any kind of insecurity, no desire to be back in hospital. One transplant patient told me that he wanted to be taken back before he even reached home; he had this feeling that he needed to be in hospital "in case anything went wrong". I have no such feeling. I believe implicitly what Maurice Neligan has told me about my surgery being very successful. I am not a cardiac cripple. I reckon I did not go through all this pain to go through the rest of my life feeling unsure, insecure. No. I suffered all this pain, this near-death, that I might be a whole person again. My recovery is a cause for perpetual celebration.

Telephone call from the Mater just now at 10 p.m..

"Bill, this is Coronary Care here. You had a blood sample taken before you went home and we have just got the result of the analysis."

"Is there a problem?" I ask, trying to hide my concern.

"No. Not really. Nothing we can't sort out. Your potassium level is a bit high. We'd like you to come in tomorrow morning, about nine, for a check-up."

"Of course. I'll be there."

My initial reaction after I put the phone down is one of near despair. Home just a few hours and things already going wrong! My wife talks to me, calms me, makes me see the incident in a totally different light. Rather than feel aggrieved, despairing, I should feel very reassured that there is such a vigilant staff at the Mater, that I am so closely monitored that nothing is allowed to go unnoticed.

❏❏❏

To the Mater this morning for the potassium test. The level is high and I am immediately prescribed medication to restore the balance. I come away feeling doubly reassured.

❏❏❏

My second night home. We go for a drink to our local, the Dalkey Island Hotel. Not for the drink *per se*, but for the wonderful sea view and the full moon on the water. I am allowed to take alcohol, in moderation, if I wish, but tonight I only want a mineral water. I enjoy it and have almost reached the end of it when I am aware of the ice cubes melting in the glass. It suddenly occurs to me that they were made from tap water. Near panic. I ring the hospital from the hotel foyer and explain what has happened.

"Should I come in? Am I in danger of infection?"

"No, Bill, you don't need to come in, and there's a very marginal chance that you will get infected from just a one-off like this. If you feel ill tomorrow, do ring us."

Again, reassurance. And a lesson to be more vigilant.

❏❏❏

The weather, for October, is very good. Balmy, sunny and dry. Good days for walking. I build my daily walk up, slowly. Starting with five minutes in the morning and five minutes in the afternoon, I am now, after one week, up to fifteen minutes twice a day. No shortness of breath, no tiredness, just a great weakness in my knees. This is slow to go away.

And the bones in my chest, the sternal bone and the ribs are very sore. But, with exercise and time, I am told all that will pass.

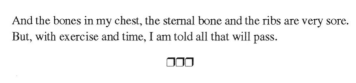

Made a new 'Will' today. God has kindly re-arranged my life this past year. I feel I must rearrange my previous 'arrangements'. Among other changes I want to have my body cremated when I die and my ashes scattered from the Baily lighthouse.

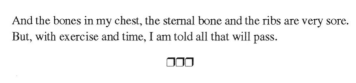

Mid-November and I am progressing very well. My knees and legs are strengthening, but the bone is still sore. I am now walking for over forty-five minutes, twice a day. And this week I felt well enough to return to work full-time. I am working on a new radio documentary, 'Heart of Grace', about heart transplantation.

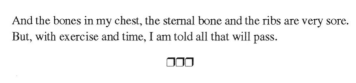

Early December. In studio at RTE for the first time in over twelve months to record some talks for 'Sunday Miscellany'. Including one which has been specially commissioned for 'Christmas Miscellany', to be broadcast on Christmas Day. The brief was to write about "What it's like to have a new heart for Christmas".

The camera comes into studio to record my first working session.

With one week to go to Christmas the old collie, Pepe has reached the end of his road. Had to have him put down today. No hope, with all the effort in the world, of improving his quality of life. A great pall of sadness on the household.

This year I can truly celebrate Christmas. Unlike last year, when I was building to the first of the many heart attacks that were to plague me until I got my new heart.

Mid-January 1995. A visit to Glencree to *An Doire Buicheas* (The Oak Wood of Thanks), where oak trees have been planted by grateful recipients and their families, to commemorate the donors and to say "Thanks!". What an appropriate place for such a wood, here in the great glen that runs from Sugar Loaf mountain to Glencree village. *Gleann na Craoi* (The Glen of The Heart).

This glen has always been one of my favourite places, especially so now. As I go up the winding hill-road out of Enniskerry village, the January sun is warm. The Sugar Loaf, like a miniature Matterhorn, guards the seaward end. And, looking west, just under the rim of the Featherbed is the village of Glencree, the gaunt, grey, scattered remnants of the old buildings stark against the brown mountain. There, in the lee of a great cliff, the German dead, from two World Wars, rest forever in the little German cemetery, under their rows of tiny, granite crosses as the mountain torrent thunders past into the gorge. This is where Synge wrote his lines, 'To The Oaks of Glencree'; the giant, immemorial oaks that, like the mountains, ring the village round:

> *My arms are round you and I lean*
> *Against you, while the lark*
> *Sings over us, and golden lights, and green*
> *Shadows are on your bark.*

◻◻◻

Early February 1995. The Saturday before St. Valentine's Day. The Annual Commemorative Mass attended by heart transplant recipients and their families and the families of the donors. It is held in the Mater Hospital Chapel. I read one of the Lessons and my grandson, John, helps take the Offertory gifts to the altar. A most moving occasion that leaves me quite speechless with emotion.

◻◻◻

I am a guest on 'The Sunday Show' on radio, a pre-Valentine's Day programme; the presenter, Andy O'Mahony, asks me what difference a new heart has made to my love life. He says, "Has it changed your attitude to women?" "No," I say, "I was always a romantic, and still am. But it has done something else for me. I was lucky enough to have been born with a built-in shit-detector. Well, after sixty-odd years of use, the detector gets a little rusty. A new heart has changed that. Has sharpened my perceptions. Given new sensitivity and range to the shit-detector. I used to be able to detect the stuff at half-a-mile, now I can smell it a mile away!" At the break in the programme, a lady rings in to express her horror at people making fun of such a serious subject as heart transplant. I answer her on air in the second half of the programme, by saying, "Madam, it's my heart!"

□□□

St Valentine's Eve. The wheel has, indeed, come full circle. This very day, one year ago, after the first of my heart attacks, I was discharged from St. Vincent's Hospital, for what was to be a very short visit home. On that day I wrote in this journal: *"But now, pain-free, albeit weak, going home, the sight of the lighthouse raises my spirits, and I make a quiet resolve that, the transplant over, I will go back to the Baily, climb the seventy-odd steps to the top of the tower again, and look westward as the sun drops behind the lovely-ugly, smog- besmirched city skyline..."*

And here I am, standing at the top of the tower on Baily, with my good friends, the Principal Keepers John Noel Crowley and Peter Duggan. Though I did have some doubts as to whether my still weak legs would make the climb. Indeed, when I rang Baily to say I was coming, I joked about my ability to climb.

"Better have a breeches buoy rigged up, or be prepared to carry me up yourselves!"

Neither was necessary. But, this evening there is no smog over the city and the big, red, winter sun slips down through a clear sky behind the serrated skyline. The afterglow suffuses the whole western sky and the water of the bay turns white.

I visit my old livingworkrooms, where some of my things are still untouched. Books and notes and a small portable typewriter. In the cupboard some bottles of wine and a half-consumed bottle of Crested Ten. On the walls just one painting. A lovely, delicate miniature of some wind-blown trees on a hill, given me by a friend when I was writing *Bright Light, White Water* here, two years ago. In my bedroom the bed is still dressed and my clothes are folded neatly in the little tallboy, reminding me of how ordered a life I lived here once, in another time, in another country of the mind. Perhaps some day I shall return to write another book here. Who knows? It is enough for me that I have made it this far, and have kept the will to go on...

□□□

Before I leave the lighthouse I go out onto the balcony and watch the sea. The ceaseless ebb and flow of the white water. And, watching it I think of what Havelock Ellis called, 'The Dance of Life'. For I am convinced now that the art of living is based on rhythm; based on cut and thrust, ebb and flow, give and take, light and dark, life and death. Life is all about surrender and vulnerability. Leaving oneself open. Abandoning oneself to the ebb and flow. Accepting, without pre-condition, *all* the aspects of life: the good, the bad, right and wrong, 'yours' and 'mine'. Life has to be celebratory, life has to be conciliatory; otherwise it is not life. And it all begins with throwing away the safety-nets so many people think they cannot do without. Rather, the first thing the dancer in this 'Dance of Life' must learn is how to relax, how to abandon. And that is difficult because relaxation and abandonment mean surrender, full, unequivocal surrender. So life is all about being totally vulnerable, totally open. Life is all about having the virtues of our faults and the courage of our gifts.

The last light has left the sky now and the sea is dark, its surface creased here and there by a thin wind blowing out of the west. Above me the great lantern spins in its bath of mercury, the powerful light revolving endlessly, part of the 'Dance of Life'; part of the celebration.

THE END